Kalashatra Gov

TANTRIC ECSTASY

THE WAY OF SACRED SEXUALITY

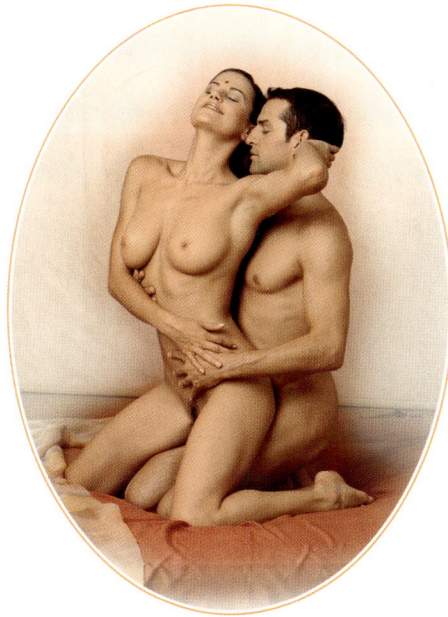

STERLING PUBLISHING CO., INC.

New York

Contents

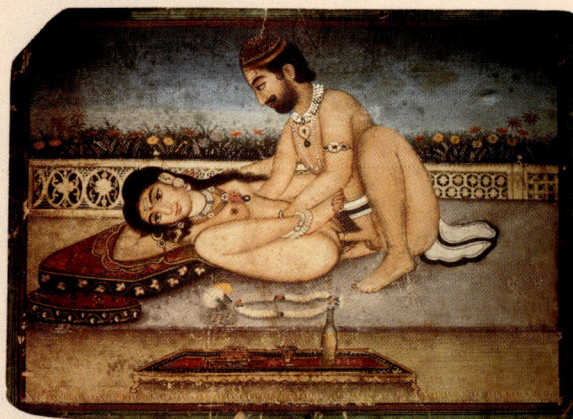

The ritual of sexual intercourse with a partner in Tantra leads to an ecstatic exchange of energy.

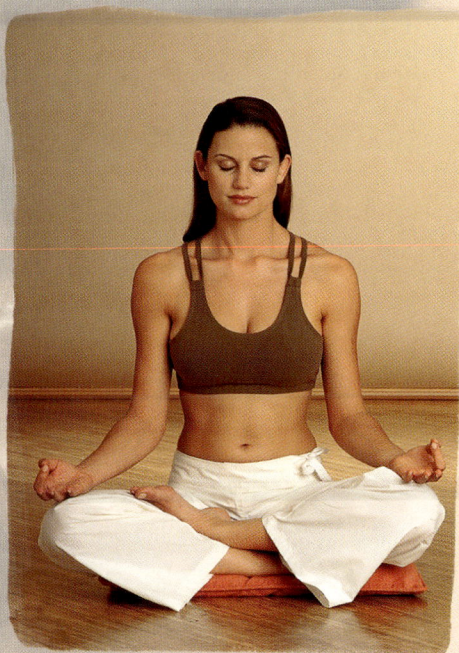

Yoga exercises can help you leave everyday life behind, find peace and contentment, and also allow time to reflect on yourself.

Time for Sensuality

Create the mood for a romantic encounter with your partner by establishing intimate and erotic rituals that enhance the ambiance.

Tantric Intercourse

Among the many tantric positions possible, you are sure to find one that is especially enjoyable for you and your partner.

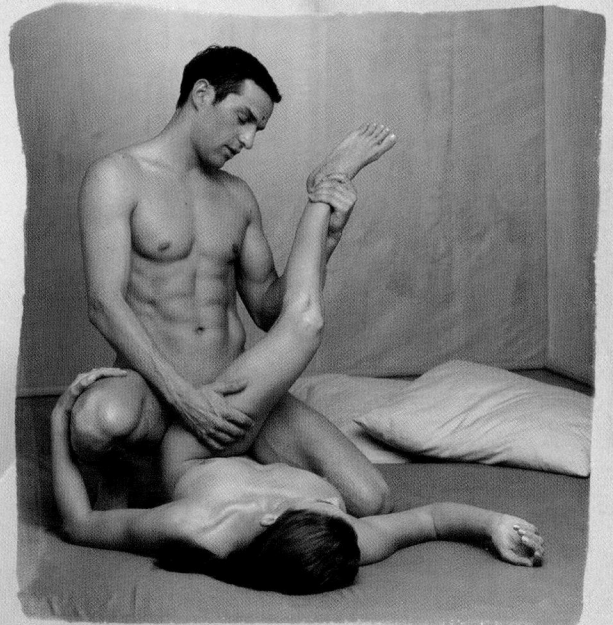

Tantra helps you develop the capability to give yourself over totally and completely to desire.

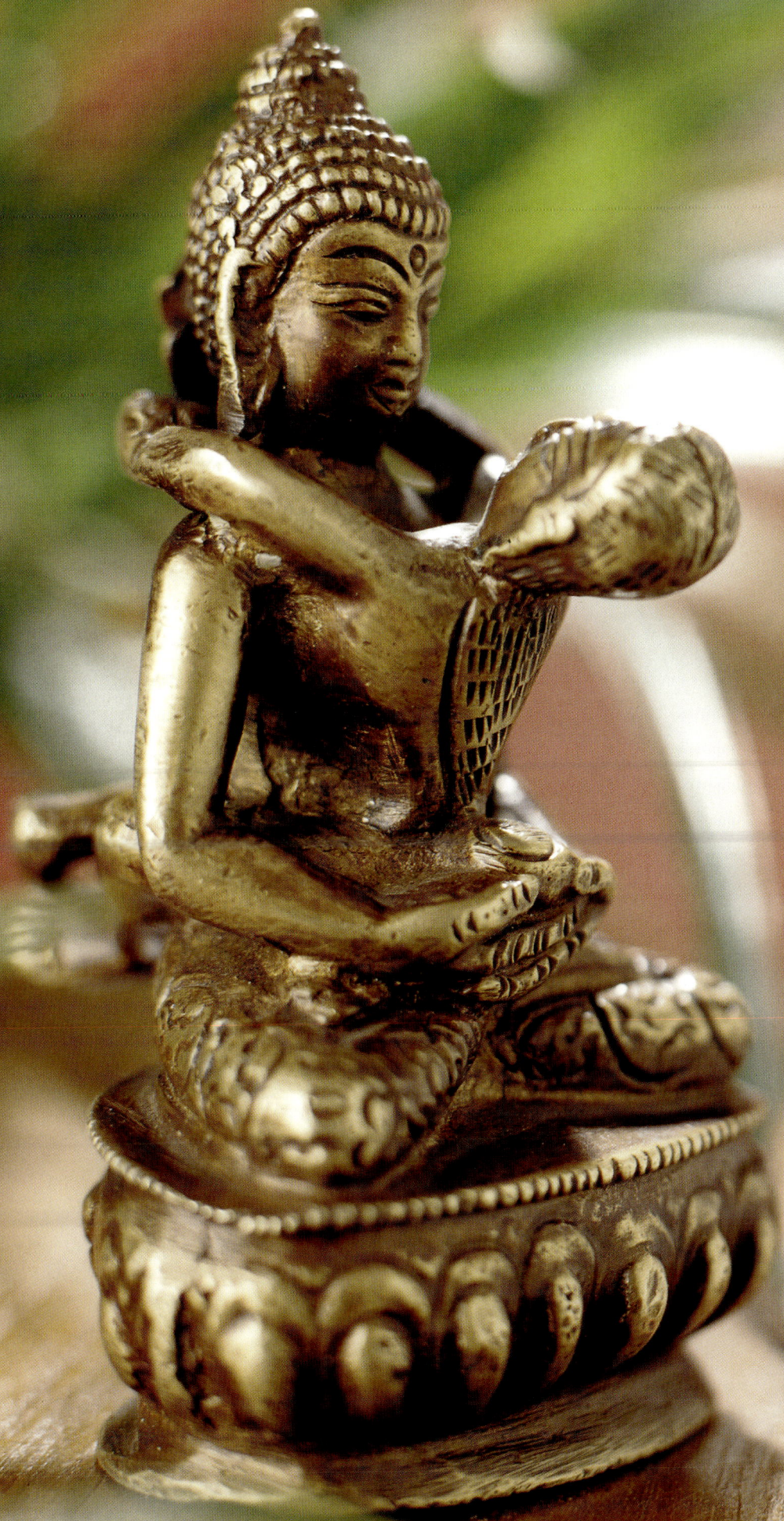

Introduction

Tantra—the "great school of sexual intercourse"—is popular today as never before.

No wonder, for Tantra shows the way to a more sensuous and positive life and sexuality, and also helps you escape the trap of casual sex.

Along with complete sexual satisfaction, trainees of Tantra learn to know the spiritual dimension of sexuality. The goal is to discover partnership in a new way, to develop trust and devotion, to reduce inhibitions, and to gain insight into the unknown peaks of ecstasy. Tantra is a balm for love, a restorative that brings new energy to every relationship.

What Is Tantra?

Tantra brings body, spirit, and soul into harmony, an integration that can help you on the path toward enlightenment. In addition, Tantra can teach you how to increase your sexual energy and acquire the high arts of love.

Tantra is an ancient Indian discipline, highly esoteric in character, that encompasses all aspects of life. Among its many topics, it examines the sacred knowledge and practices of sexuality that can be used to transform sexual intercourse with your partner into a deeply spiritual experience.

Tantra may have originated in the East, but it has the ability to enrich the lives of all the world's people, independent of culture, religion, or the time in which they live. Tantric practices can help you feel more zest for living and, naturally, more sexual pleasure while simultaneously teaching you about the deeper nature of partnership and love.

Love and Sexuality

Tantra has the ability to bring about positive change, particularly in your love life.

🔄 Your life will be altogether more colorful, insightful, and satisfying.

🔄 You learn to say yes unreservedly to life, desire, and love.

🔄 You will become more sensitive and aware, more intimately responsive to yourself and your partner.

🔄 You will learn to heighten your sexual energy, thereby increasing potency.

🔄 You will discover sensuality, develop trust and devotion, and experience unexpected peaks of ecstasy.

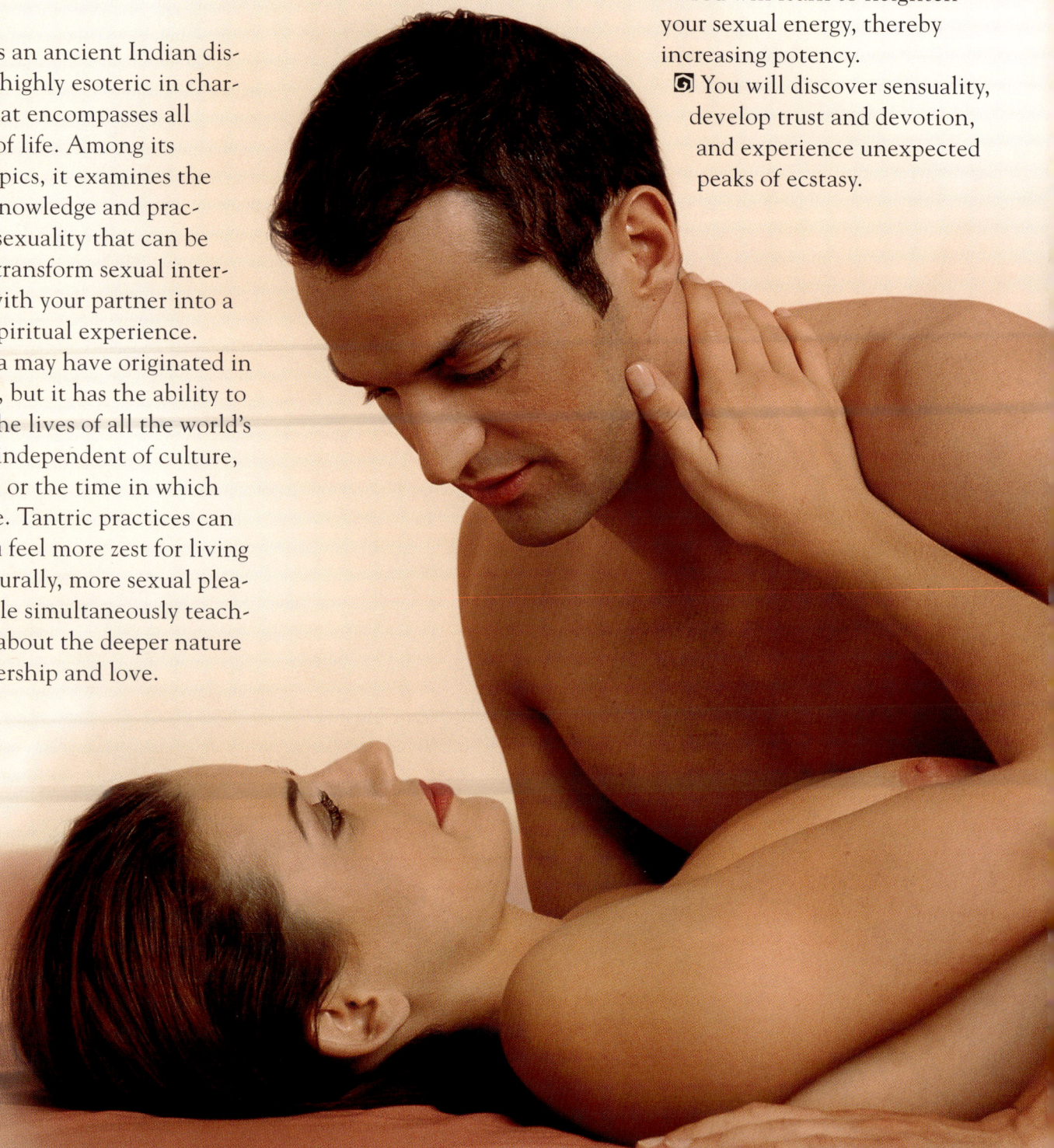

🔟 You learn to overcome anxiety and inhibition, and to resolve sexual barriers or other problems.

🔟 The quality of your sexual experiences will improve greatly.

🔟 Last but not least, tantric techniques, known as Tantra-Yoga, will help you maintain the harmony between body, spirit, and soul, which is very beneficial for general health.

How This Book Will Help You

On the following pages, you will learn the essential elements of the art of love and discover how the practice of Tantra can be utilized to awaken your sensuality and sexual pleasure.

A brief background in the Indian arts of life and love will be provided, illustrating how erotic massage, touch, and sensuality can help you cultivate tenderness and greater sensitivity toward your partner. In addition to historical information, you will be given specific instruction about Tantra-Yoga. Through body postures, breathing techniques, and meditation, you will learn how to prepare for sexual encounters with your partner while simultaneously increasing your vitality.

This book will also acquaint you with the secrets of orgasm, the possibility of retaining sexual energy, and how to improve the functioning of your chakras.

Classic tantric positions and special sexual techniques that serve to enhance the spiritual nature of love will be described in detail, guiding the way to ecstatic and enlightening experiences. Finally, you will also find suggestions about the selection and use of stimulating aphrodisiacs obtainable from health food or natural healing stores.

In using this book, please consider that Tantra is primarily intended to help you become a more spiritual and philosophical individual, but you should use the contents as a foundation for personal experiences and experimentation! Do not get lost in thinking of the "correct" technique; rather, discover your individual Tantra by allowing yourself the space needed for personal development. The only qualifications are a relaxed frame of mind as well as spontaneity and intuition. Therefore, follow the offered suggestions, techniques, and instructions in a playful and flexible manner and do not hesitate to adjust them to your needs.

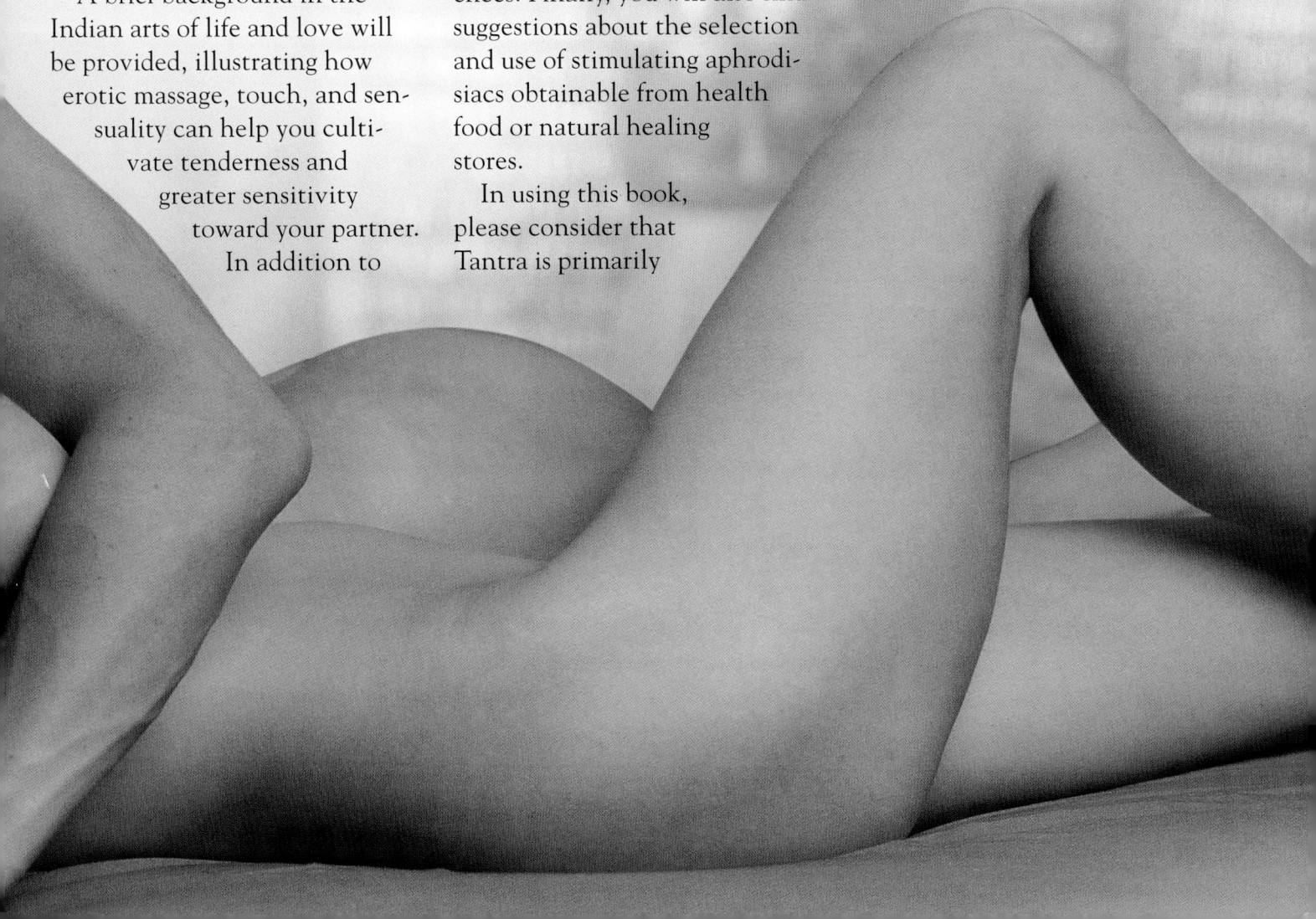

What You Should Know About Tantra

The term Tantra comes from the Sanskrit word meaning "thread" or "woven fabric" and also encompasses the meaning "inner nature" or "essence." Initially, a series of esoteric rituals and scriptures from the spiritual world of Hinduism and Buddhism were combined, developing into what we now know as the Tantras.

The Hindu scriptures document the dialogue between Shiva, the male deity, and his beloved Parvati, who is the personification of Shakti (see page 16). In esoteric-philosophical conversations, Shiva describes the rituals of Tantra to his partner. In these

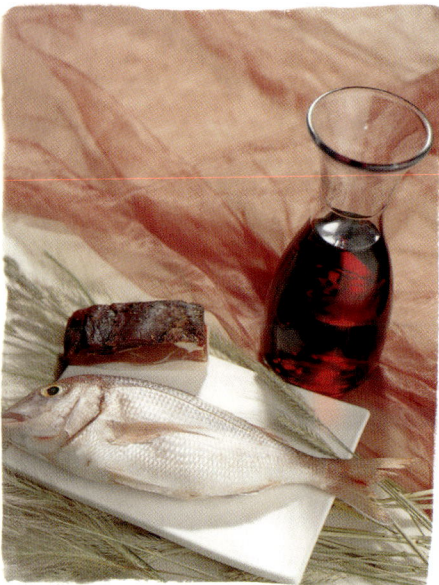

According to tradition, wine, meat, and fish symbolize tantric pleasure in life.

discussions, the five "M's" are of especial importance: *maithuna* (sexual intercourse), *mada* (wine), *matsya* (fish), *mansa* (meat), and *mudra* (grain). All are symbols of the joy and sensuality of life that explain why Tantra is described as the spiritual way of joyous living.

History and Origins

We know little about the origins of Tantra, but the initial source of tantric ideas probably dates back more than 10,000 years, when the rise of matriarchal-based culture first appeared. Archaeological discoveries of sexual symbolism give tangible evidence that tantric rituals emerged very early within Indian culture in the form of fertility and mother cults. These rituals, it is certain, were handed down orally from generation to generation for centuries.

Search for Unity To some extent, Tantra also played a role in the Upanishads, the 2,500 year old holy writings of Brahmanism. This text describes Hindu creation, in which the longings of the female deity create a unification of polarities, resulting in the creation of man and woman. Evidence of tantric ecstacy is seen in the ruins of Indian temples: they depict the sexual

encounters between male and female deities as an expression of this search for unity.

Equality After the fifth century A.D., Tantra had a considerable influence on Hinduism and Buddhism. Counted among the best known Tantras are the Kularnava, the Ananga-Ranga, and also the Kama Sutra, which was composed from twelve different writings by various authors around the fourth century A.D. The adherence to ritual and study found in the Kama Sutra and other Tantras went against the authority of the orthodox Vedic scriptures primarily by ignoring the caste system and declaring all individuals equal but also by the inclusion of orgiastic rituals that followers dared practice only in secret.

Between the sixth and seventeenth centuries, Tantra reached the height of its popularity in Assam and Bengal. Many Brahman communities, particularly the Buddhist cult of Vajrayana, which developed from Mahayana Buddhism, united with Tantra and utilized the practices for themselves. Buddhist Tantra was then further developed in Tibet and, in turn, influenced Hindu Tantra.

Taoism was also influenced by tantric thought. China's Taoists were already well acquainted with tantric doctrine over 2,500 years ago, at which time it circulated throughout all of China and Nepal; today, the classical form of Tantra is mostly associated with northern India.

While it has taken longer to become known in the West, Tantra is now a familiar discipline and seminars have become widely available.

Goal of Tantra

Although there are many different schools and varieties of Tantra, the goals are usually very similar. Analogous to a master key that can open many doors, Tantra has the ability to unlock different treasures and make them accessible.

Ultimately, it depends on you. Would you like to use Tantra solely to maintain your health, or would you rather achieve *samadhi*, enlightenment?

Harmony The primary concern of Tantra is the harmonic development of human potential whereby soul, spirit, and body are attended to in order to maintain health. Therefore, Tantra says yes to sensuality and yes to the often disparaged carnal sex because, to the practitioner of Tantra—a tantrician—there is no separation of flesh and spirit. Everything that life offers is holy! Tantra values the human

Tantra develops all the senses. They are all required for a life of meaning.

body as a divine desire-giving gift, for without desire there is no procreation, no development, and no evolution. The only sin acknowledged by Tantra is to do harm to oneself or other people; such actions violate the tantric reverence for life and damage the spiritual values within people.

Today, Tantra offers a unique opportunity, not only because it emphasizes acceptance of desire, pleasure, and the body, but also because it seeks to develop a conscious relationship with physical desire that is directly opposed to salacious, casual sex.

Tantra offers practitioners a release from mechanical, short-term appeasement and also relief from many sexual problems and disorders. Impotence, erectile dysfunction, difficulty with orgasm, guilt, performance anxiety,

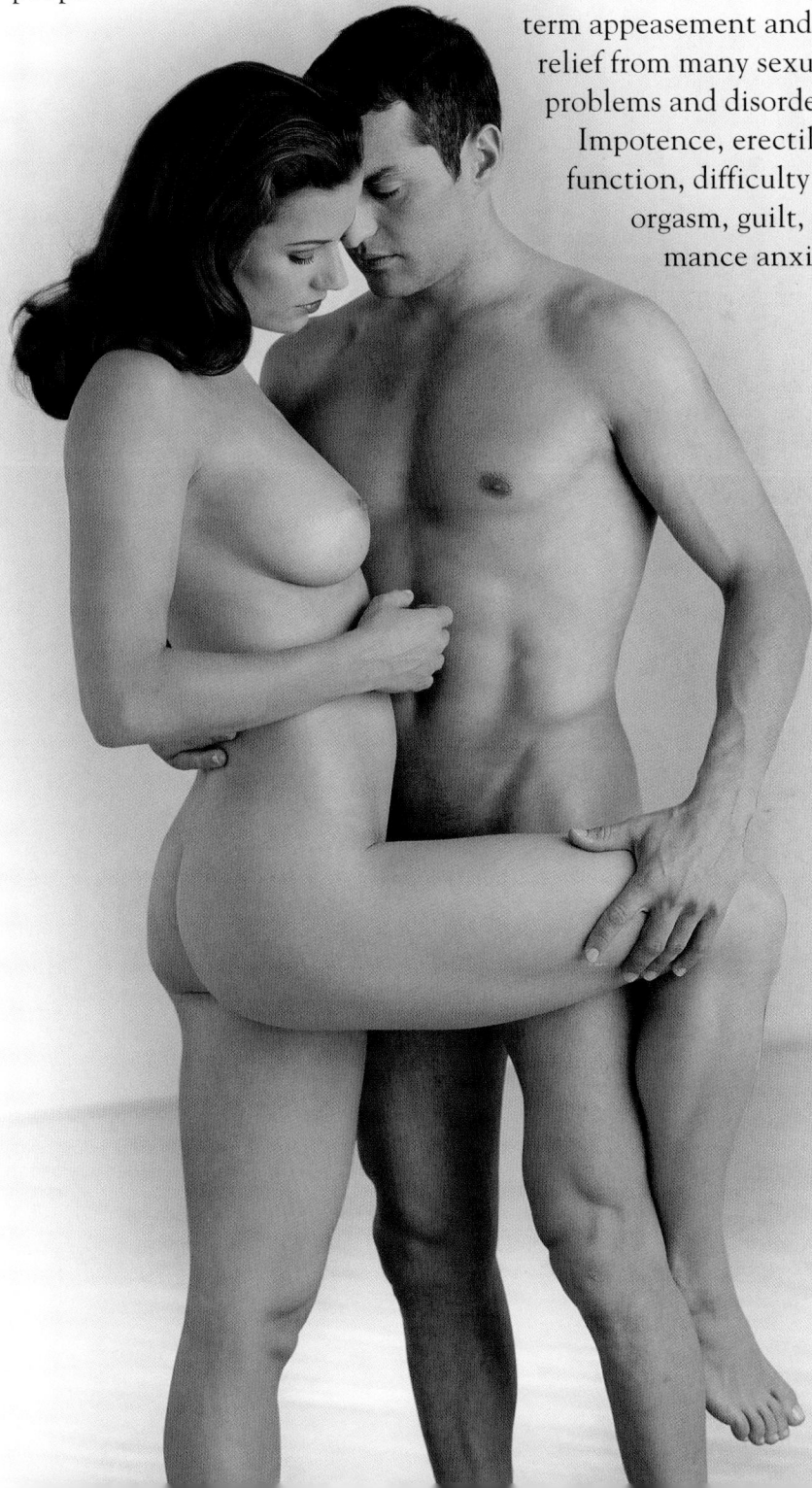

and inhibitions are often caused by false ideas about morality, lack of contact with one's own body, or emotional blocks. All these problems can be overcome with Tantra.

Tantra is not about directly confronting sexual problems you may have; rather, the goal is to forget your inhibitions completely and practice the lessons of Tantra instead. Should you have problems reaching orgasm or suffer from so-called frigidity, attempting to surmount the problem or feel more during intercourse will only make these goals even more difficult. The same applies to overcoming erectile dysfunction. Erectile dysfunction is very rarely caused by surgery, medication, or other organic factors; the trouble is most likely caused by anxious concentration directed at maintaining an erection.

Enjoy Relaxation

Tantra provides the possibility of erotic encounters focused on relaxation and openness, not the pursuit of erection and orgasm. An emphasis on performance usually has a negative impact, and Tantra is about joy and acceptance. Along with a healthy diet and lifestyle, as well as the avoidance of toxic substances, Tantra promotes a series of specific techniques from which all organs of the body, especially the genitals, can profit.

Ultimately, Tantra strives to improve both the functioning of sexual organs and, more important, the expression of eroticism and a heightening of orgasmic capability. This is not something achieved through willpower. These goals are easily accomplished by understanding and practicing tantric techniques.

Expansion of Consciousness To utilize all one's energy resources, to make the act of love more passionate, and to open your chakras—these are only steps on the path leading to the main goal of Tantra, which is also know as the Yoga of love.

Both Tantra and Yoga pursue no less a goal than the expansion of consciousness and attainment of bliss. In contrast to the ascetic-oriented Yoga, Tantra places importance on the attainment of ecstasy. Sex viewed as the veneration of the abstract (the godlike) in tangible form (the beloved) increases unity and expands love. This occurs through Transcendence—exceeding the borders set by conventional experience.

Individuals can expand their everyday, routine consciousness into one in which they experience bliss and enlightenment—otherwise known as *samadhi*. As the differences between male and female, or you and me, are gradually dissolved, a sense of unity is created, comprised of love and attentiveness. Tantric sex is not possible without this merging and the gentle affection it produces.

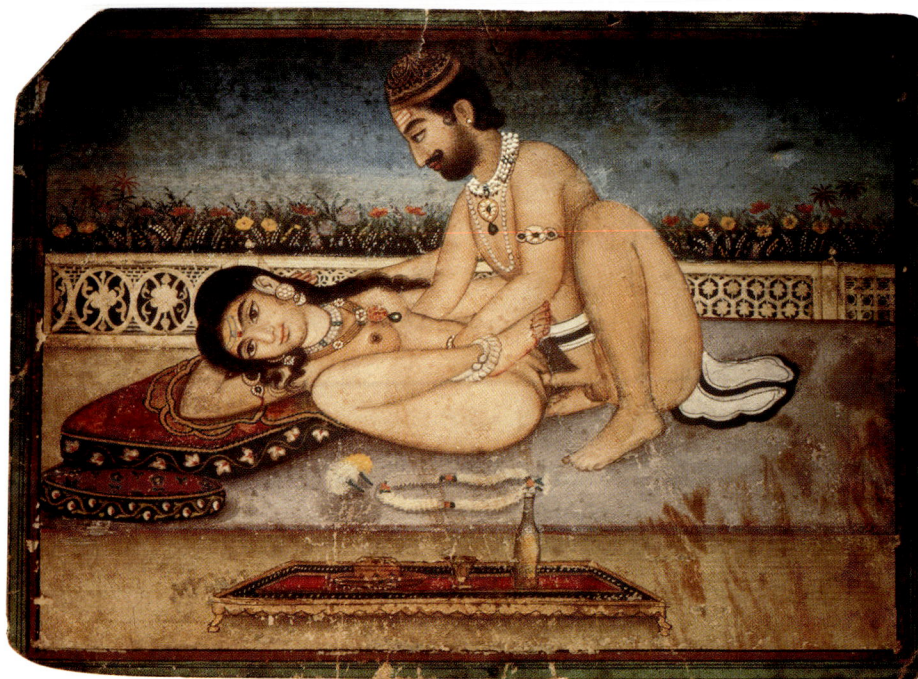

In ancient tantric tradition, sexual intercourse between man and woman is always the main goal.

The Way of Tantra

Healthy, fulfilling sexuality, spirituality, and transcendental love are the most important goals of Tantra. But how can they be attained, and what techniques would be used?

Although each school of Tantra uses its own methods to achieve these goals, techniques that are developed usually follow rules observed by all forms of Tantra.

To begin with, Tantra does not follow the path of asceticism, unlike nearly all other spiritual disciplines that have their origins in Hinduism or Buddhism. The basic tenets of Tantra—belief in sensuality and acceptance of all life—reject all forms of self-abnegation as a senseless and futile struggle against human nature.

Pleasure Through Renunciation

If an individual rejects life, sexuality, and sensuality, liberation will be difficult to achieve. Therefore, Tantra refuses to reject emotions such as desire, passion, and pleasure, believing it is more productive to incorporate them into the discipline. Nevertheless, Tantra does not promote the reckless expression of sexual urges.

Without control of sexual energy and without patience and concentration, a grasp of the sanctity of the sexual act is not possible. Seen in this light, Tantra also has its ascetic side; it is only through the renunciation of casual sex that an individual can reach the peaks of ecstasy.

Along with the inner principles regarding joy of life and the spiritual aspect, definite methods also play a role within Tantra.

◎ Sensuality depends the senses of taste (wine, certain food), smell (aromatic oils, incense), and touch (stroking, tender massage).

◎ Sexual intercourse becomes ritualized with the use of classical love positions.

◎ A technique of relaxation encourages tranquility and an anxiety-free, meditative, erotic experience.

◎ Control of sexual excitement and orgasm will prolong the sexual encounter.

◎ Through Tantra-Yoga and breathing exercises, sexual energy will be stimulated, body awareness will be enhanced, and the chakras will be further developed.

◎ Mantras (holy incantations) will be employed.

Finding Individual Variations

Essentially, every individual must find his or her own form of Tantra. Throughout the course of time, many forms of Tantra have developed, depending on the era, country, or predominant culture. The original form of Tantra practiced in medieval India, for example, could not be practiced today without complications.

Tantra offers you new possibilities, but the methods should always be adjusted to your needs. The techniques in this book provide a foundation for modern Tantra that you and your partner can experiment with. Together, you can discover which methods are especially appealing—to express your sensuality, strengthen your sexual energy, and most importantly, to experience meditative unity.

Trust and tender affection are as important to tantric sex as technique.

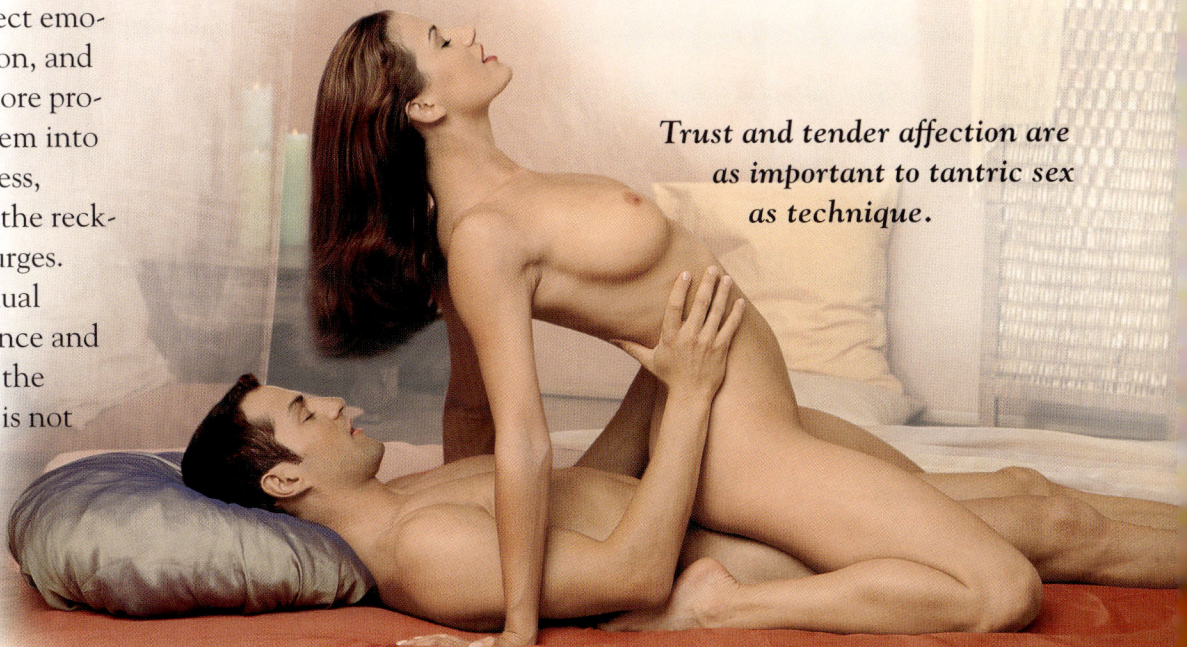

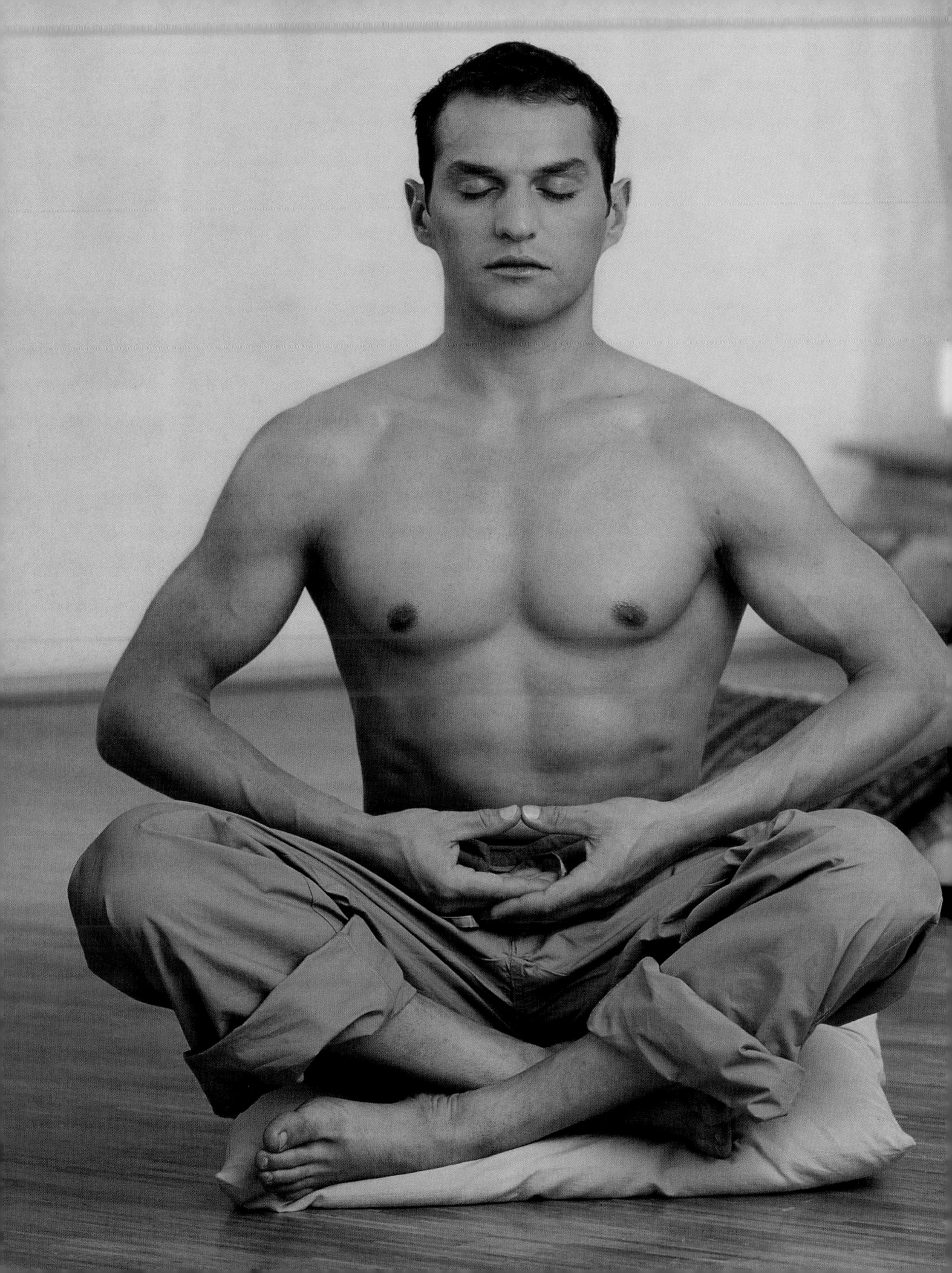

Esoteric Foundations

For a full understanding of Tantra, it is necessary to examine its esoteric background. Unfortunately, a superficial view often confuses Tantra with sexual gymnastics, but the deeper meaning of the Eastern love arts can only be found by expanding the closed borders of the consciousness of self. Tantra exercises activate the flow of energy to the astral bodies, which in turn help develop the chakras, the points of spiritual energy in the human body.

Tantra also focuses on the conception of reality that is hidden behind the external web of illusory appearances. This allows students of tantric exercises to see themselves and their partners anew, with attentive and loving eyes.

The Origin of Tantra

In order to better understand the framework of Tantra and the purpose behind the duplication of certain techniques, it is valuable to know something about its background and underlying esoteric precepts.

The following pages will use concepts taken from the Sanskrit such as Shiva, Shakti, chakras, or kundalini, but this does not mean that the practices of tantric lessons are connected with a specific religion. In its modern form, Tantra can be used by anyone, independent of culture of origin or religion! However, in this book many of the original terms will be retained since they convey the important principles of Tantra that might otherwise be mistranslated.

The tantric worldview assumes the existence of a powerful cosmic force that is the underlying basis of all life and in which spirit and matter are united. Therefore, despite the many deities in Hinduism, divinity is actually seen as indivisible energy. Tantra makes no distinction between the worldly and the godly, because the *Brahman*—the omnipresent reality or universal soul—is found everywhere. All beings, without exception, feed from this cosmic energy.

The tantrician finds the ultimate truth in meditation as well as in sensuality—or better still: in meditation about sensuality!

Individuality Tantra is a system of ideal monism, meaning that only one ultimate principle is the foundation for all phenomena; therefore, Tantra supports all life in its complete abundance.

Tantric training advances the belief that the godlike is present in all living creatures, a tenet that should be realized by every individual; unfortunately, most people create self-imposed restrictions that stand in the way. Tantra tries to break the chains of these limitations, hence the root *Tan* of Tantra is similar in meaning to expansion or extension.

The use of both tantric techniques and the rituals of sexual intercourse will help to expand your self-awareness, making a

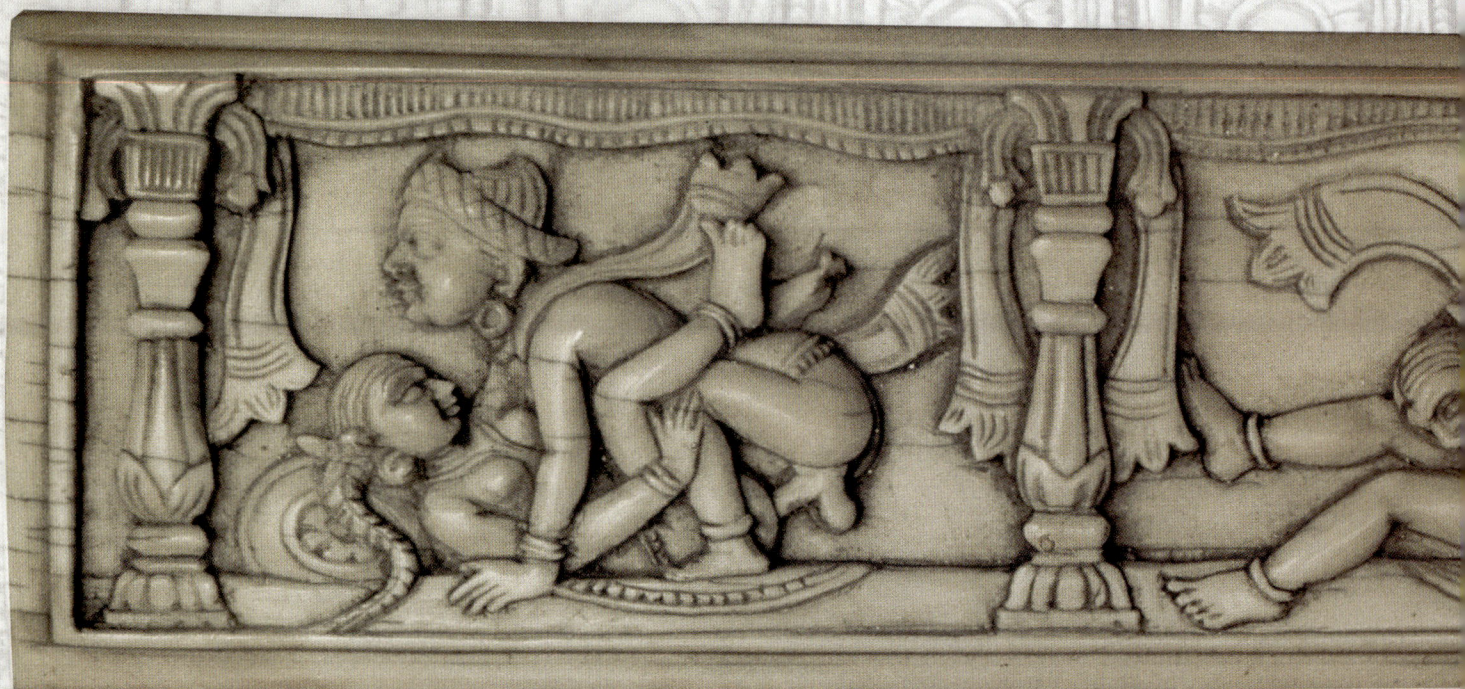

return to your cosmic origins possible.

The Traditional Source

The Hindu story of creation reveals much about the philosophy of Tantra, which worships the female as the source of all that exists. According to the sacred texts, the original female god was responsible for animating the energy source that created the universe, including heaven, earth, oceans, rivers, fish, birds, and all other animals.

Although the goddess was at first filled with happiness at her creation, she eventually became aware of a feeling of emptiness. This suggested that, despite her handiwork, she was bored and somewhat lonely in her godly isolation. That is why she ultimately began to create humans, producing the female form as her first effort! This was so pleasing that she took this form for herself as Kali, and then created a male who entered the world in the form of the god Makahala.

It is believed that mankind was created through the tantric intercourse between Kali and Makahala. That is why ecstatic love play between the two gods is often the central theme in tantric art.

Unity of Man and Woman

Tantra assumes that man and woman form an inseparable union. Any supposed separation is merely the consequence of an illusion that originated when humans first became incarnate and the self became separated from its divine origins.

The longing for a return to divinity is reflected in the eternal search for the opposite sex, which is a more or less instinctive desire for interaction and unity that exists in all people. Sexual stimulation and intercourse are the ultimate goals of desire—the purpose is to restore the original physical and spiritual union.

It is therefore most important for those who practice Tantra to rise above the ego-consciousness and self. To achieve this, sexual intercourse must serve as a ceremonial rite whereby transcendental awareness is intensified and one's lover acquires a much more meaningful role than mere sexual partner. The male represents a vital embodiment of the everlasting male principle, the god Shiva, while the woman is transfigured into a living symbol of the goddess Shakti, the sensual personification of Parvati.

Numerous works of art portray intercourse between man and woman.

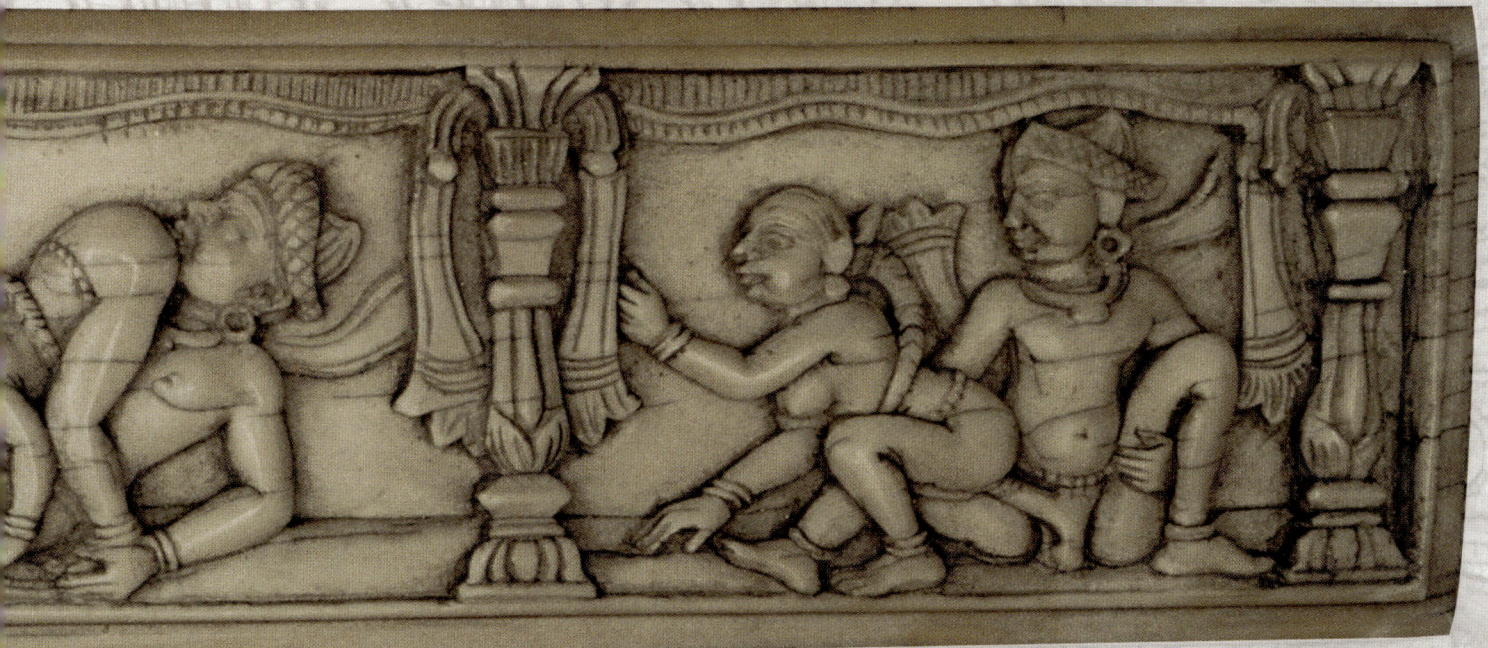

Shiva and Shakti

In Tantra, the deities Shiva and Shakti personify the male and female poles. Shakti corresponds to the moon's energy, otherwise known in Chinese cosmology as Yin, while Shiva is equivalent to the energy of the sun, known as the Chinese Yang. Similar to Yin and Yang, Shiva and Shakti complete each other through eternal interaction.

Shiva

Shiva (Sanskrit for "gracious") is the personification of male energy and, alongside Vishnu and Brahma, is one of three main deities of Hinduism. Known also as *Sundaresh-vara* (beautiful man), *Bharaiva*

(the terrible), and *Mahadeva* (great god), Shiva is venerated as the all-powerful ruler who is considered the supreme yogi and also master over death. Shiva also represents the principle of discovery and awakening, which can be further interpreted as absolute awareness—which is located in the uppermost chakra of the body (see page 19).

Shiva is often depicted as the cosmic dancer Nataraja, whose dance represents the continual changing of the universe, however, in Tantra he symbolizes sexuality and the erotic. Shiva plays such a large role in both Hinduism and Tantra because he is the embodi-

ment of the everlasting male principle.

He is often shown together with a cobra or oxen that serve as riding mounts. Some depictions show Shiva with a drum and trident, others as a curly-haired god meditating on a tiger-skin rug and wearing a wreath of snakes and skulls.

Shakti

Shakti (Sanskrit for "power") symbolizes the female pole of the Hindu sacred triad. She represents the everlasting female principle, the great goddess who activates all cosmic energy through intercourse with the male deities. In Tantra, it is assumed that women have essentially more Shakti available than men, and indeed, no male god can survive without his Shakti, his female energy that is personified in the form of a divine consort.

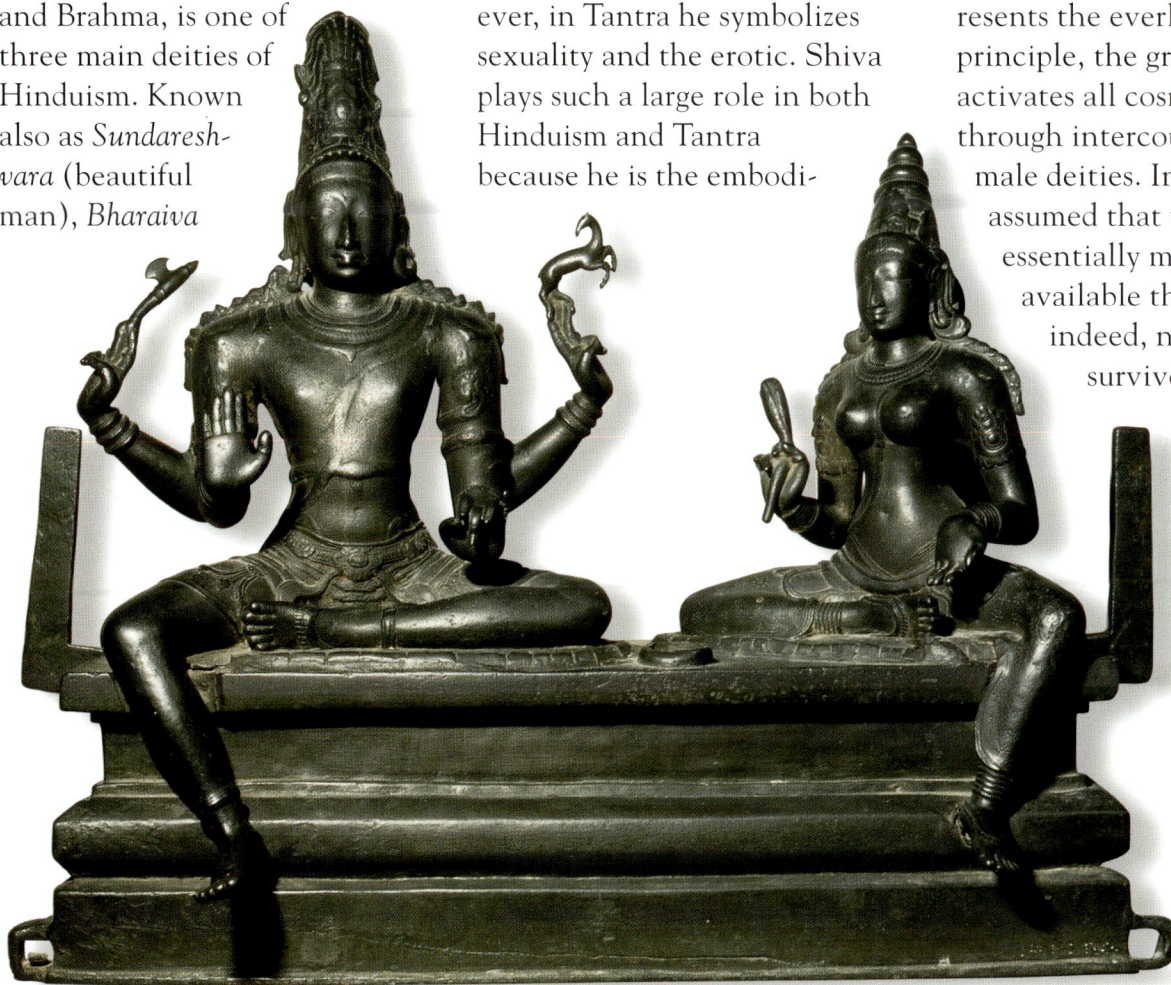

Both Shiva and Shakti play an important role in the mythology of Tantra.

Shakti's opposite poles have two differing personifications—one as the loving and sensuous Parvati; the other as Kali, the fierce goddess of destruction who is usually associated with the Divine Mother of the Universe.

She also symbolizes the Principle of Vitality, which stimulates all matter and creates nature. The astral bodies form the lowest chakra at the point of Shakti energy, located at the base of the spinal column (see page 18).

Yin and Yang, Shiva and Shakti—this attraction between male and female is reflected in Tantric philosophy.

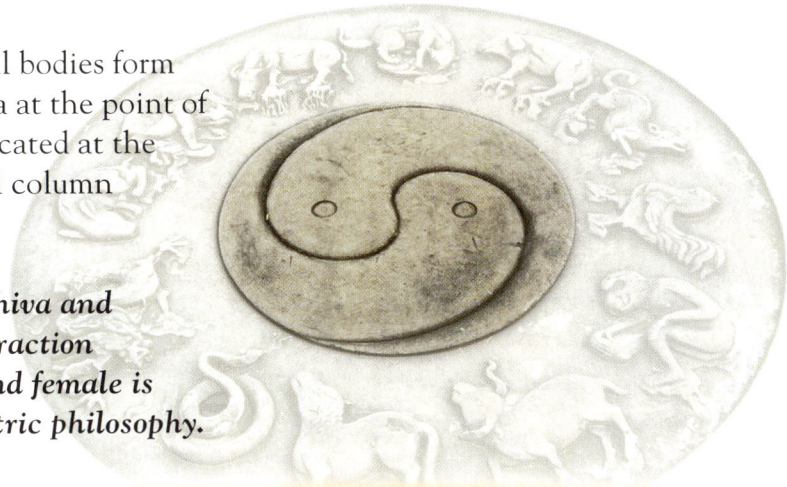

Kundalini—The Power of the Snake

The practice of Tantra is founded upon the mysteries of the male-female union of energies. What is generally called enlightenment—or *samadhi*—is the personal consciousness of the union between Shiva and Shakti. While Yoga provides the individual an opportunity to experience this union, Tantra reaches toward understanding together with a partner.

To accomplish this, Tantra neophytes learn to stimulate the life force (Shakti) and combine it with cosmic knowledge (Shiva). The process of this awakening is accelerated through Tantra and is reflected in the image of kundalini.

Kundalini is both a representation of cosmic energy and of Shiva, and is depicted as a coiled snake that rests at the base of the spinal column in the body. Specific tantric exercises known as Kundalini-Shakti awaken the energy which then rises along the spinal column, activating all other chakras on the way. This leads to strong health and a fulfilling life. Similar to

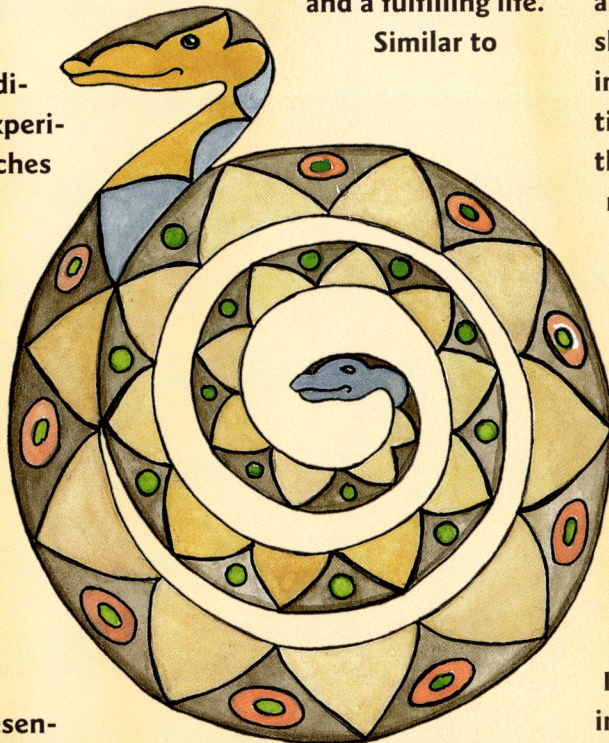

Yoga lessons, tantric techniques support the activity of the chakras. Chakra is a Sanskrit word meaning "wheel" or "whirling." Chakras are not physically or anatomically established organs, but points of energy and consciousness in the human body. They are aligned along the spinal column and shine within the body, influencing organs and glandular functioning as well as emotions and thought. All spiritual development corresponds to an awakening of the chakras.

It is also possible to influence individual development through deliberate stimulation of certain chakras. Tantra is especially concerned with activation of the lower chakras (root and sacral centers) that influence sexual energy. The short overview on pages 18 and 19 introduces the most important aspects of the chakras such as related colors, symbols, and mantras. In addition, the overview presents h the physical and mental functions that a specific chakra influences.

The Chakras

Muladhara Chakra
Root center

Color Red
Mantra LAM
Symbol Square
Location Perineum, base of the pelvis, coccyx
Meaning Survival, source of energy, preservation
Area of Influence Urinary system, kidneys, adrenal glands, colon, rectum, bones, and coccyx
Positive Aspects Vitality, determination, self-preservation, perseverance, rhythm, ties with nature, trust, and grounding
Negative Aspects Selfishness, indolence, oversexed, existential fear
Physical Disorders Colon, bladder, and kidney disorders, prostate problems, bone disease, constipation, high blood pressure, anemia
Emotional Disorders Fear, mistrust, physical weakness, decreased libido, masochism

Svadhisthana Chakra
Sacral center

Color Orange
Mantra VAM
Symbol Crescent
Location Sacrum, abdomen, area above the genitals
Meaning Sexuality, reproduction
Area of Influence Gonads, genitals, abdomen, sacrum, and pelvis
Positive aspects Passion, libido, creativity, vitality, body awareness, attractiveness, healing energy, potency
Negative aspects Overly emotional, sexual addiction, coercion, aggression
Physical Disorders Venereal disease, painful menstruation, prostate disease, impotence, low-back pain, blood and lymph disorders, skin disease
Emotional Disorders Weakness, frigidity, depression, animosity toward life

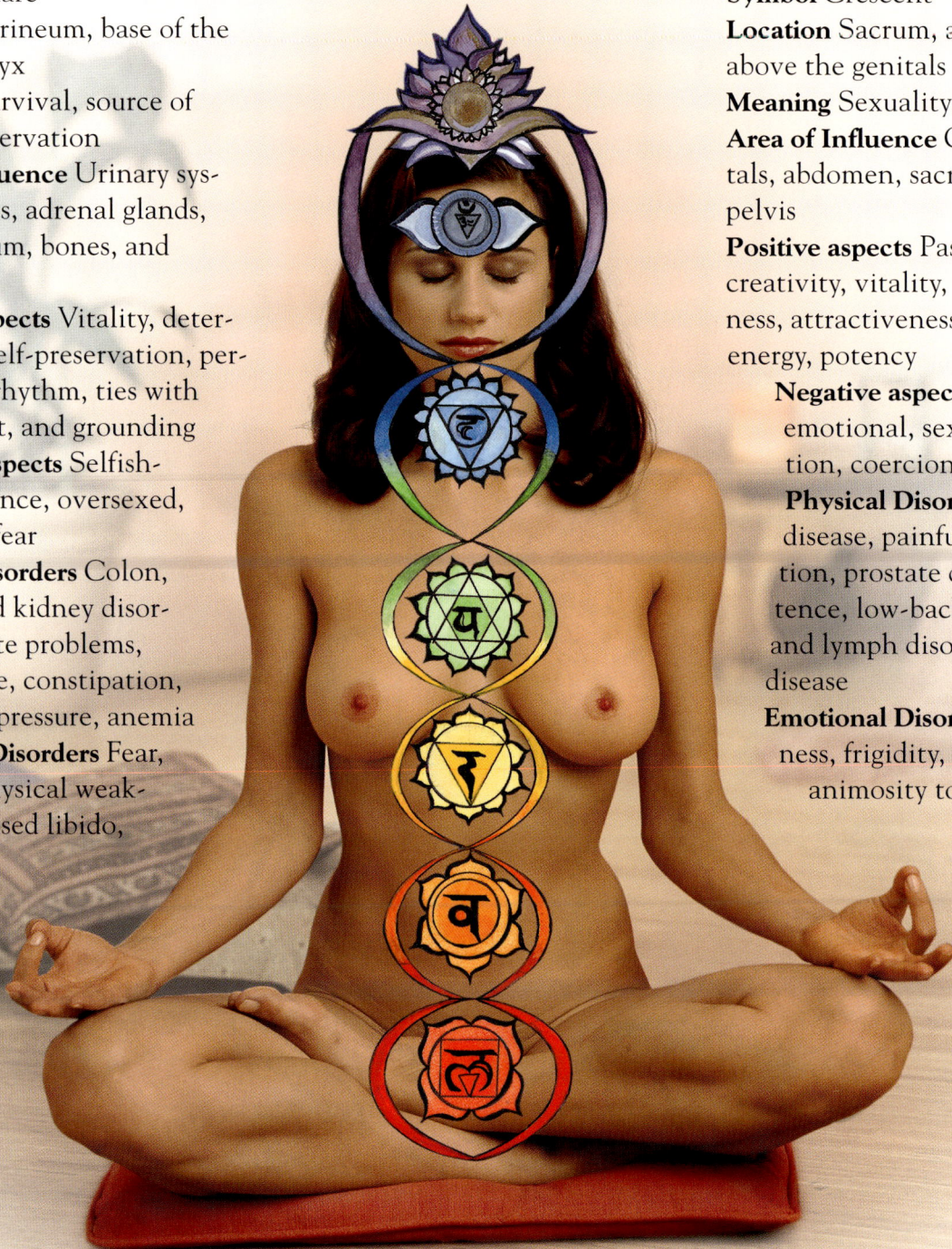

Manipura Chakra Solar plexus center

Color Yellow
Mantra RAM
Symbol Triangle
Location Stomach, lumbar vertebrae, solar plexus, upper abdomen
Meaning Emotions
Area of Influence Liver, pancreas, abdominal cavity, spleen, stomach, gall bladder, autonomic nervous system
Positive Aspects Sympathy, sensitivity, emotions, persistence
Negative Aspects Sentimentality, coldness, self-pity, obsession with power
Physical Disorders Stomach problems, indigestion, weight problems
Emotional Disorders Fear, rage, irritability, sleep disorders, nightmares

Anahata Chakra Heart center

Color Green
Mantra YAM
Symbol Hexagon
Location Breastbone, heart region, middle of the chest cavity
Meaning Love, humanity
Area of Influence Heart, blood, circulation, thorax, thymus gland
Positive Aspects Love, warmth, communication, artistic expression
Negative Aspects Arrogance, egoism, unkindness
Physical Disorders Heart trouble, high blood pressure, lung disorders
Emotional Disorders Unsociability, isolation, coldness, loneliness, fear of being alone

Vishuddha Chakra Throat center

Color Light blue
Mantra HAM
Symbol Circle
Location Larynx, cervical vertebrae
Meaning Mental energy and communication
Area of Influence Thyroid gland, throat, jawbone, voice, larynx, windpipe, respiration
Positive Aspects Ability to communicate, harmonic self-expression, ability to discriminate, individuality, good language and tone
Negative Aspects Intolerance, thirst for glory, unrealistic, overemphasis on the intellect
Physical Disorders Pain in the neck, teeth, throat, and shoulder, illness in the laryngeal region
Emotional Disorders Timidity, inhibition, confusion, fear of isolation

Ajna Chakra Third-eye center

Color Dark blue
Mantra KSHAM
Symbol Circle with two wings
Location Between the eyebrows, middle of the brow
Meaning Intuition, wisdom
Area of Influence Pituitary gland, cerebellum, face, eyes, ears, nose, sinuses
Positive Aspects Self-awareness, creative energy, intuition, integrity, spirituality, inspiration, soulfulness
Negative Aspects Selfishness, self-aggrandizement, power hungry, egoism
Physical Disorders Stomach pain, migraine headaches, brain disease, eye trouble, impairment of the sense organs
Emotional Disorders Poor memory, weak concentration, feeling of futility, fear

Sahasrara Chakra Crown center

Color White, violet
Mantra OM
Symbol Lotus blossom
Location Top of the head
Meaning Spirituality, spiritual knowledge of the world
Area of Influence Middle of the brain, pineal gland, eyes, whole organism
Positive Aspects Oneness with the universe, intellectual power, spirituality, piety
Negative Aspects Black magic, detachment from world, seclusion, lack of ego
Physical Disorders Headache, chronic illness, weak immune system
Emotional Disorders Spiritual depletion, no joy of life, depression

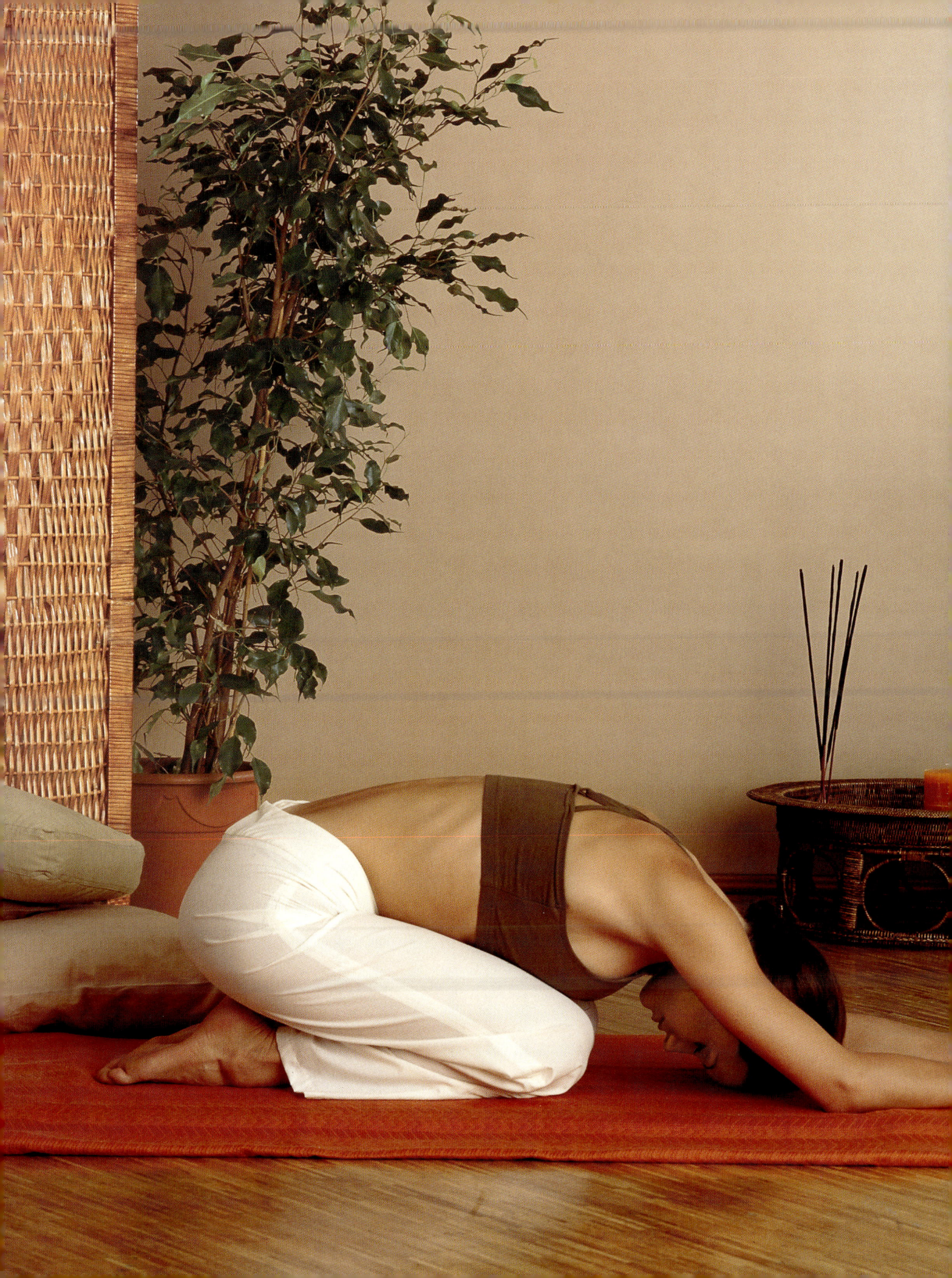

Tantra-Yoga

Entry into the tantric arts begins with Tantra-Yoga. These are exercises comprised of special relaxation techniques, yoga positions, breathing exercises, and meditation. The brief program of exercises offered here serves to heighten sexual energy and strengthen the pelvic area while simultaneously keeping the body healthy, vital, and flexible.

The training also provides you with the tools needed to reduce stress and eliminate inhibitions and fear. Debilitating emotions such as these quickly ruin the experience of pleasure in lovemaking and prevent the expression of true feeling between partners. Practitioners of Tantra-Yoga further benefit by learning how to accept themselves and their sexuality unconditionally.

What Is Tantra-Yoga?

Yoga and Tantra have essentially the same goal: to harmonize body, spirit, and soul and to guide the way to illumination.

Tantra focuses primarily on the ecstatic sexual relationship between man and woman. However, before practicing the lessons together, there are some techniques that each partner should perform alone. The following exercises help to prepare you both physically and mentally by:

🔊 Boosting your sexual energy
🔊 Helping you to know and love yourself better
🔊 Keeping your body flexible and healthy
🔊 Purifying and therefore harmonizing the body, allowing you to know yourself better
🔊 Activating the chakras

Before you try traditional tantric positions, it is suggested that you have at least one month's experience with the following Tantra-Yoga exercises. In the event that you and your partner would like to begin simple tantric instruction immediately, suitable exercises in sensuality and erotic massage are also offered (see page 60).

What Does Tantra-Yoga Do?

In contrast to Yoga, which promotes the inward direction of all energy and concentration, Tantra seeks to develop extrinsic spirituality and awareness, especially between you and a partner. Nevertheless, both Yoga and Tantra are ultimately pursuing the same goal: the great liberation, otherwise known as *samadhi*.

Tantra-Yoga seeks to bring both the individual and communal aspects together in harmony, for it is highly important to learn awareness and to know your level of energy: only then will it be possible to give your partner the intense concentration that Tantra exercises require.

Tantra-Yoga techniques are specifically, but not exclusively, directed toward activating sexual energy and raising consciousness. The purpose of the techniques is to unite the male and female poles—

Shiva and Shakti—into our sexual awareness, transforming the sexual act into a sublime ritual with profound spiritual effects.

Tantra-Yoga Practice

Tantra and Yoga originate from the same source, yet they diverge in practice: Yoga emphasizes asceticism while Tantra stresses ecstatic pleasure. The following lessons should express the combined elements of both disciplines and incorporate inner concentration as well as joy and ecstasy. Enjoy the Yoga positions and breathing exercises in the mindset of Tantra—concentrate, but without stress or pressure: do not force yourself!

Prepare a pleasant atmosphere in advance by using scented perfume, color, or candles, and practice with a smile on your face. This will activate healing qualities when you treat yourself with love.

Yoga lessons are also useful in massaging your partner, a technique that sets the mood for sexual pleasure.

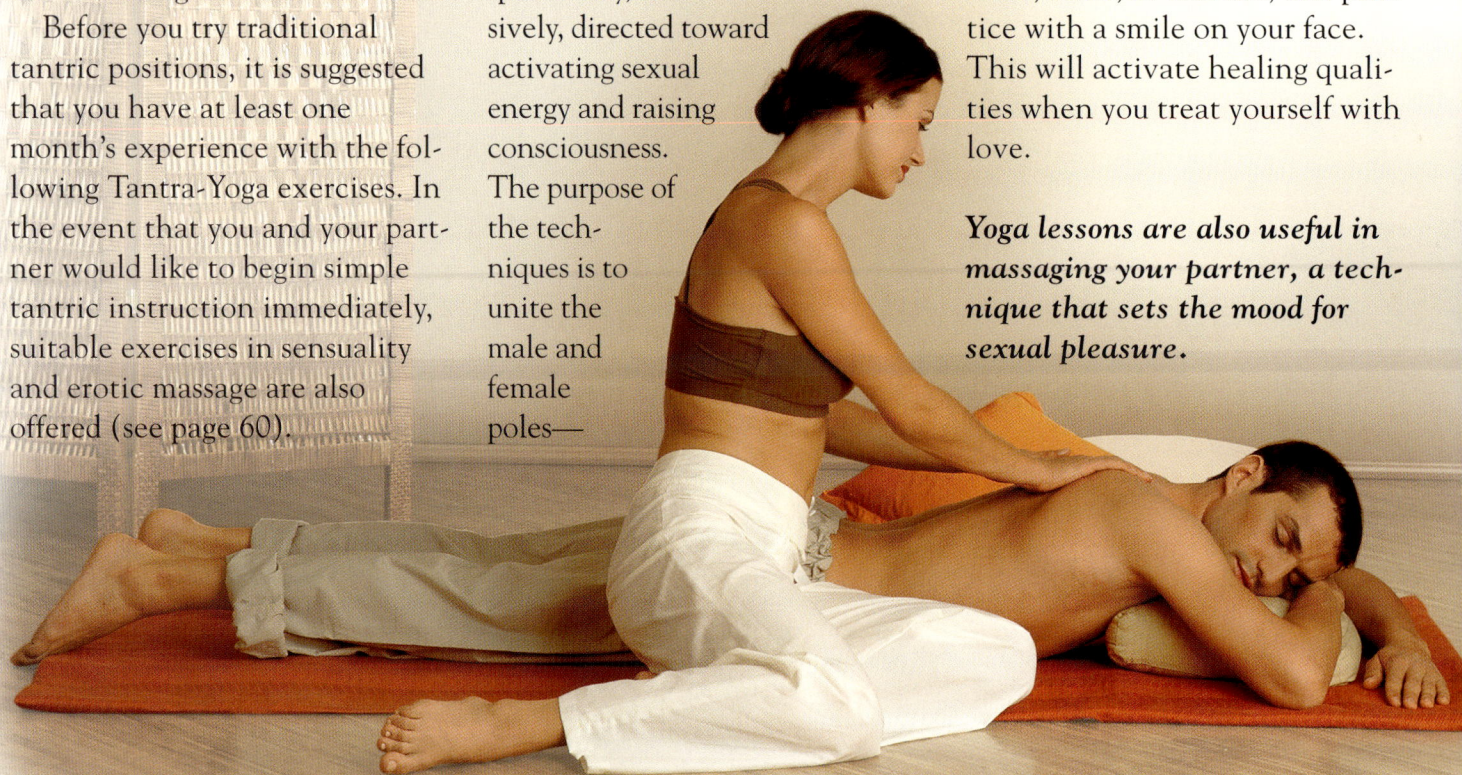

Energy and Harmony

The ability to practice meditative Tantra requires that the mind be free of everyday concerns and the body physically relaxed. Yoga lessons can help you prepare both your mind and body.

The following program of simple exercises serves to sharpen your physical awareness. They help reduce stress, overcome blocks, and stimulate life energy, all of which aid in the preservation of your health. What's more, the exercises help keep the spinal column flexible and purify the channels of the astral tubes—known in Yoga as *nadis*—which assist in counteracting many sexual problems.

The exercise program should be performed once a day at convenient times such as early morning or in the evening before you go to bed. Be sure to wear light, comfortable clothing or, whenever possible, simply exercise naked. If you use a red or orange colored covering or exercise mat, you will be able to stimulate the activity of the lower chakras (see page 18).

Always remember to warm up thoroughly by stretching, breathing deeply several times and shaking your arms and legs robustly. Never exercise on a full stomach. This is how to correctly prepare your body for Tantra-Yoga.

The Slanted Posture

Lie flat on your back with the palms of your hand lying next to your thighs. Inhale deeply through the nostrils as you bring your legs together and tighten your stomach muscles. Then press down with your hands and raise your legs straight up, perpendicular to the floor and stretch them over your head while supporting your lower back with your hands. In the final position of this posture, your legs should be together, knees straight and feet pointed slightly toward the back—but you should still able to see them. Your chin should be pressed against your chest.

Breathe gently through your nostrils, relax your stomach, and hold the position for about a minute. To release, reverse the steps, allowing your vertebrae to slowly unwind.

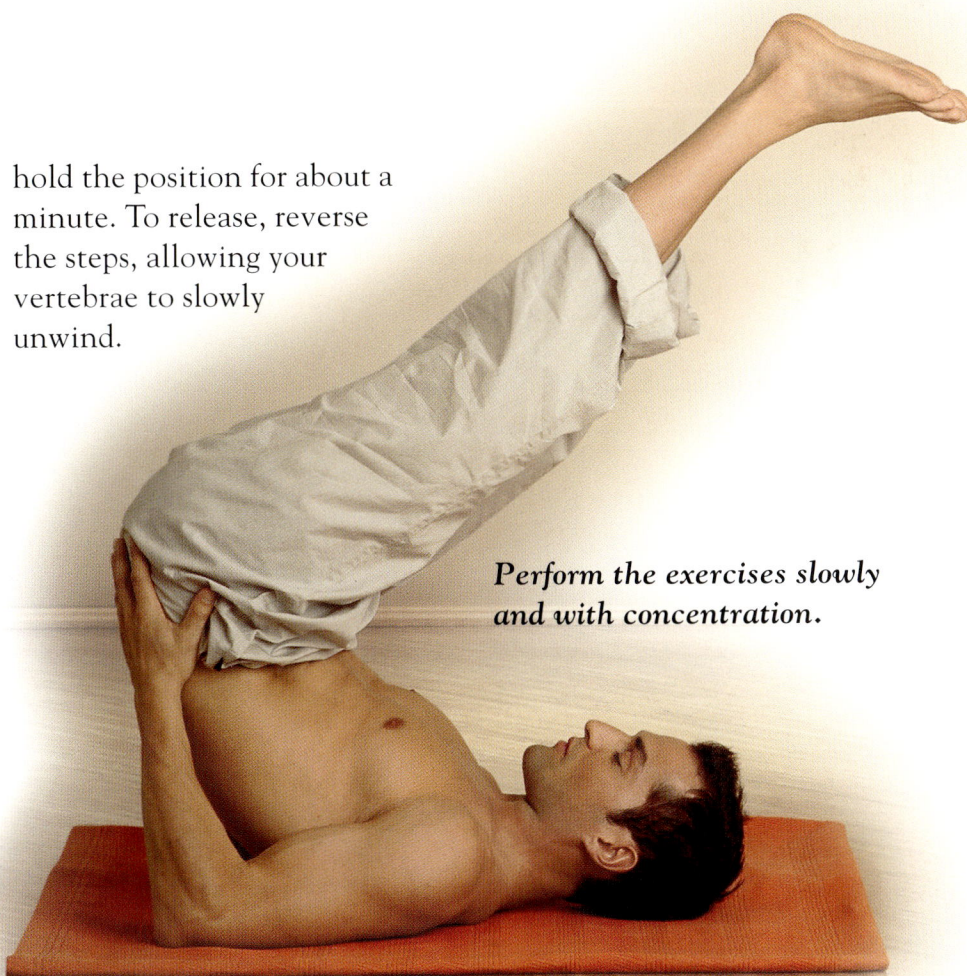

Perform the exercises slowly and with concentration.

Yoga-Mudra

The starting position is the heel posture. Sit on your heels with knees and big toes touching each other. If you find this too difficult, place a small pillow between your backside and feet. Hold your back erect and allow your arms to dangle loosely at your sides. Close your eyes and breathe deeply several times. As you exhale, let your torso sink slowly forward until your forehead touches the floor. Place the back of your hands next to your feet. Breathe naturally and be conscious of the mild pressure the movement makes against your thighs. Remain in this position for about a minute then, beginning with the lumbar region, slowly straighten up.

Yoga-Mudra helps you to relax and find tranquility.

The Grasshopper

Lie on your stomach with your legs together and forehead touching the floor. Place your arms next to your body so your hands are near your hip. Make loose fists with the thumb outside, pointing upward. Inhale deeply as you lift your right leg upward, supporting the movement by pushing your fists against the floor. Hold this position for a few seconds before slowly lowering it, then perform this motion with the left leg. Repeat this exercise three times alternating your legs while making sure your hip bone is in constant contact with the floor. At first, you may not be able to stretch too far upward—a few inches is quite enough. When finished, turn your head to the side and relax.

Repeatedly stretching and relaxing the muscles helps to strengthen them.

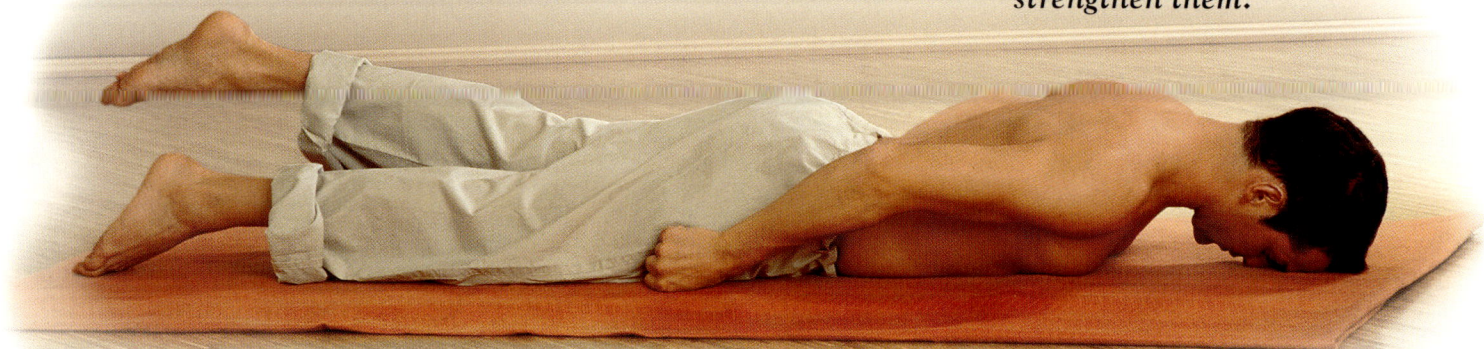

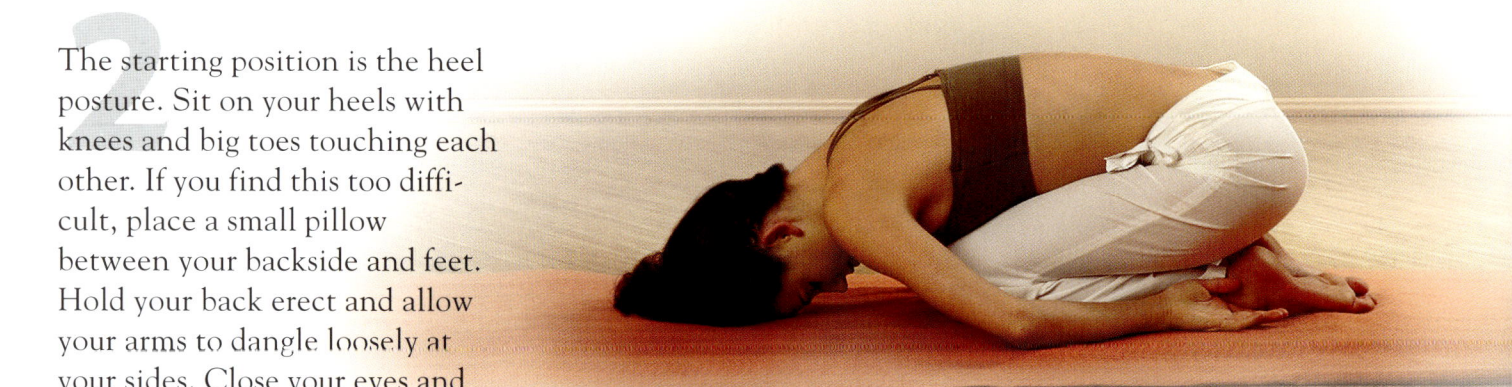

The Cobra Posture

Lie on your stomach, keeping your legs together, then turn your head so your chin is placed against the floor. Bend your arms so your palms are facing down and your elbows touch the floor. Inhale slowly and raise your head until

Doing the cobra posture correctly will strengthen your back.

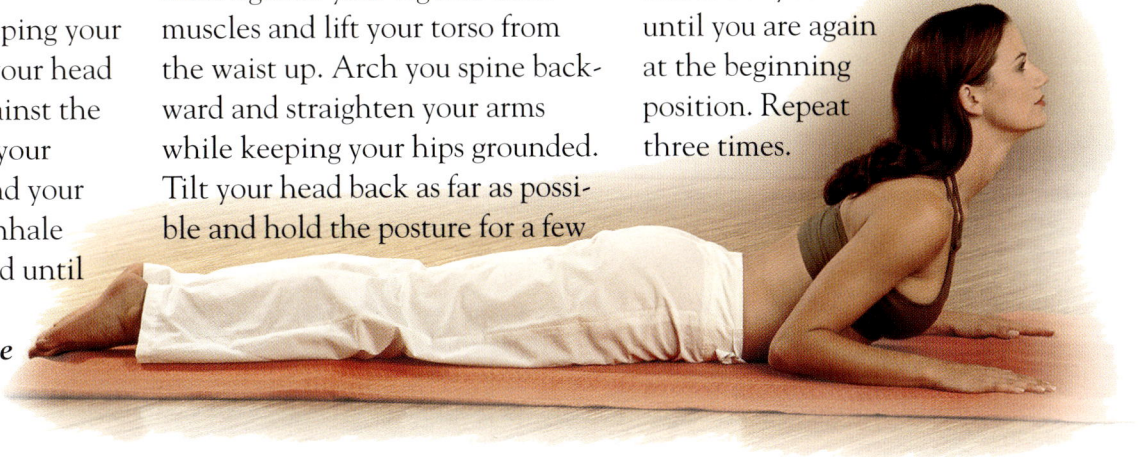

you are looking straight ahead, then tighten your leg and back muscles and lift your torso from the waist up. Arch you spine backward and straighten your arms while keeping your hips grounded. Tilt your head back as far as possible and hold the posture for a few

seconds, then relax your shoulders and lower your head and torso until you are again at the beginning position. Repeat three times.

The Crocodile

Lie comfortably on your back—legs angled, knees bent, and soles of your feet touching the floor. Extend your arms out to either side,

Make sure the knees and feet always remain together.

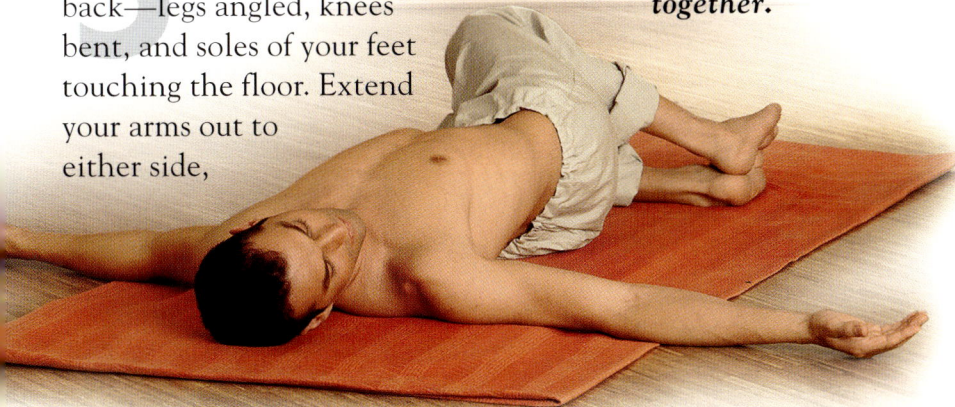

palms facing upward. Inhale slowly while turning your head to the left, letting your legs fall to the right. Rotate as far as possible without causing yourself strain or pain. Exhale while you slowly bring your head and legs back to the starting position, then turn toward the other side—head right and legs falling to the left. Repeat these movements very slowly and relax briefly between rotations.

The Tree

Stand with your feet together, back straight, and arms hanging at your sides. Concentrate on your feet. Imagine that you are deeply rooted to the earth. Shift your weight onto your right leg, then raise your left foot and place it on your right thigh, slightly above the knee. As soon as you are stable, form a ring with the thumb and index finger and stretch your arms slightly out to the sides of your body. Remain in this position for about a minute, then slowly lower your arms and your foot. Repeat the exercise with the opposite leg.

You are better able to balance if you concentrate on a point several feet in front of you.

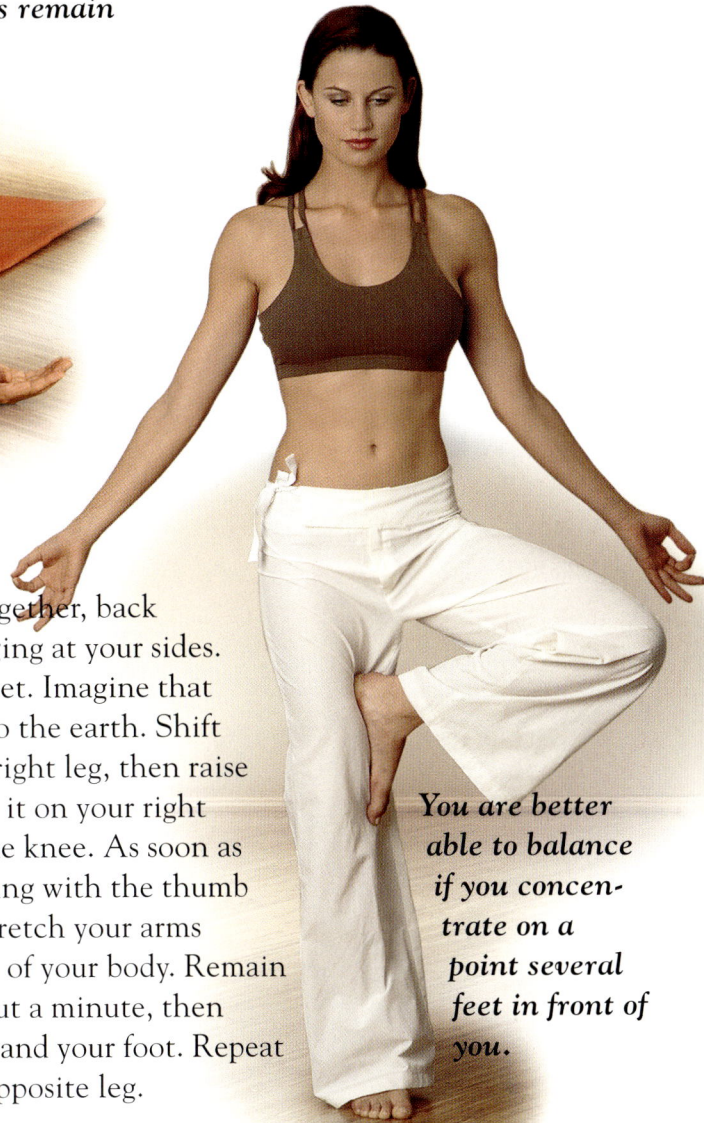

Yoga Relaxation

7 Always end the series of postures with a relaxation exercise that can be felt throughout your body. While still on the floor, become conscious of the weight, gravity, and warmth of your body. If you still sense any stress, with each deep exhalation sim- ply imagine it flowing out of your body and into the floor. Take pleasure in the relaxed immobility of your limbs and allow your thoughts to be calm. Before ending the relaxation position, you should also thor- oughly stretch your muscles and breathe deeply several times. Yoga relaxation requires only a few minutes and is especially helpful in reducing tension, which has a negative impact on sexual energy. This position should be performed regularly, especially if you suffer from sex- ual blocks, inhibition, or anxiety.

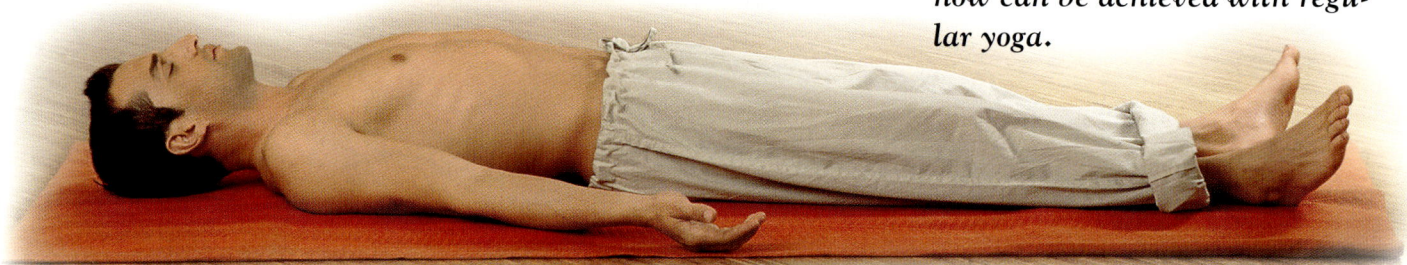

Total relaxation in the here and now can be achieved with regular yoga.

7a For the relaxation posture, lie on your back with eyes closed, then spread your legs slightly and let your feet fall outward. Your arms should lie next to your body with your palms touching the floor. Listen to your body. How do you feel in it? Now lift your right leg a few inches off the floor. Tense your foot, calf, and thigh for four seconds, then bring the leg slowly back down. Repeat this exercise three times, feeling your leg become more relaxed with each lift. Exercise the left leg.

7b Now tighten the buttocks. Hold this position of your muscles as long as it remains comfortable, then relax the muscles thor- oughly. Switch between tension and relaxation three times, or as long as you can maintain a feel- ing of well-being within the area.

Tighten different muscles one after the other.

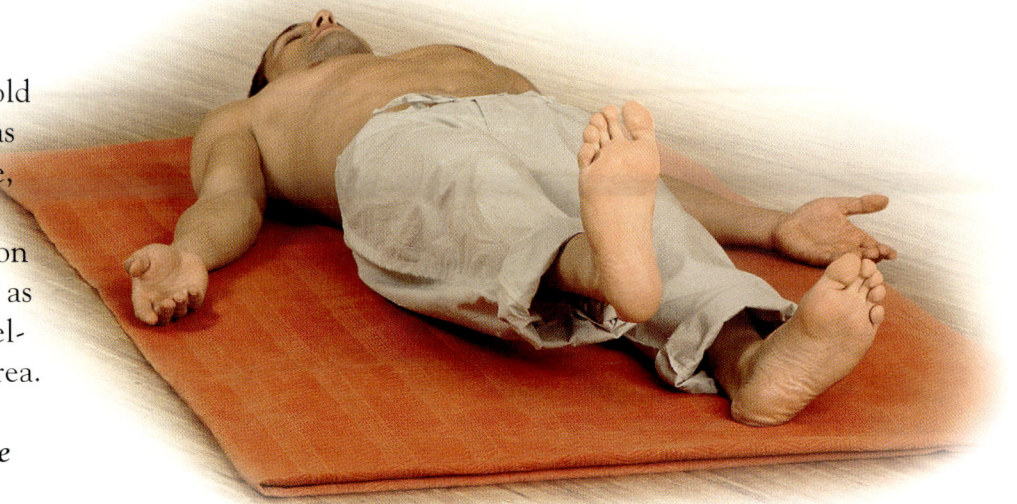

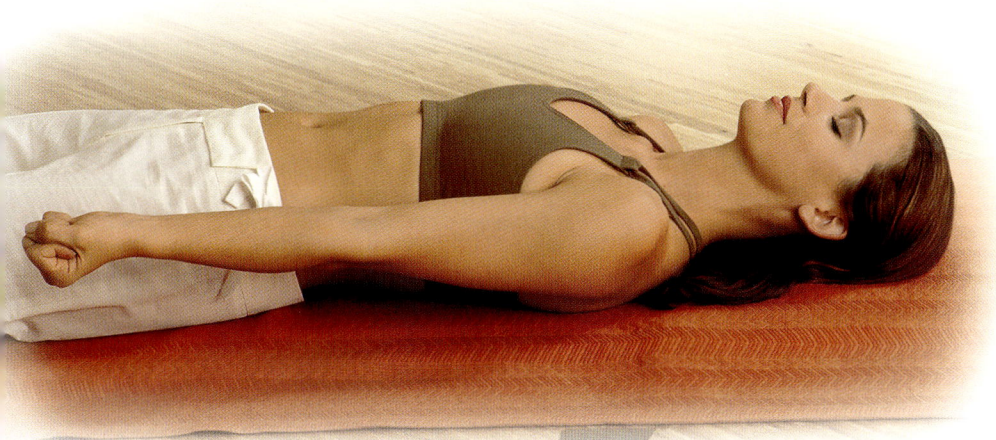

The arm muscles will also be carefully stretched. When relaxed, they will feel pleasantly warm.

7c Lift your right arm a few inches off the floor. Make a clenched fist and tighten the muscles in your forearm and upper arm. Slowly count backward from ten, lessening the tension slightly with each declining number. To do this, you must increase your exhalations, so do not forget your breathing pattern, which can also be regulated by counting. When you have reached one, open your fist and relax all the hand and arm muscles. Repeat three times, and then do the exercise with the other arm.

7d Tighten your stomach and back muscles by lying on the floor and deeply exhaling. Hold your breath for about four seconds keeping the stomach muscles tense, then slowly inhale and relax them. Repeat this three times. Now pull your shoulders upward, toward your ears; hold in position, then let them drop slowly down. Repeat this sequence of tension and relaxation three times. It is very effective against blocks in the cervical spine region and tension in the shoulders.

Lastly, lift your head a few inches from the floor and clench your facial muscles, so your face becomes wrinkled. After about four seconds, bring your head back down to the floor while relaxing your face. Repeat this exercise three times.

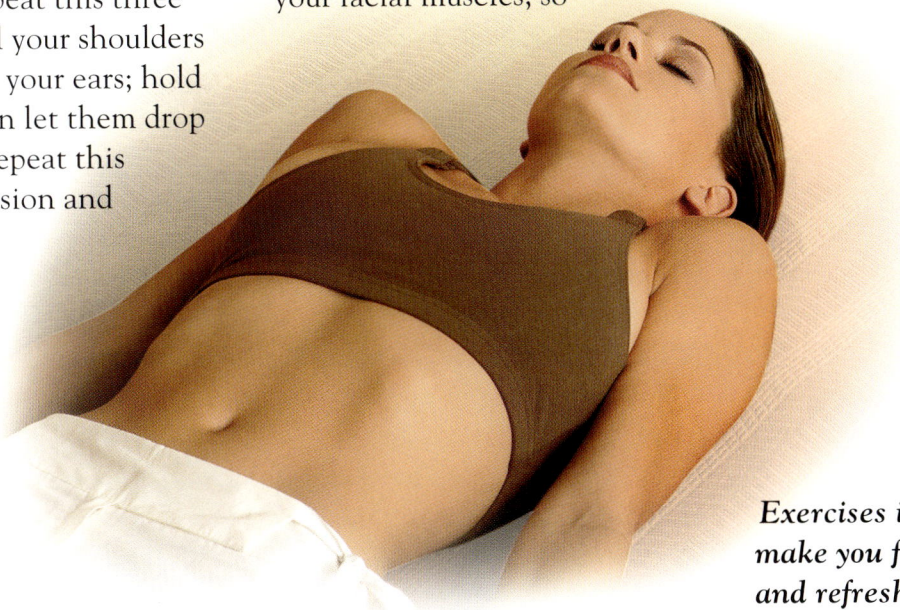

Exercises in relaxation will make you feel undeniably rested and refreshed.

How to Increase Your Sexual Energy

Tantra-Yoga has a positive effect on the entire body and is instrumental in activating the chakras, which play an important role in sexuality.

The following Tantra-Yoga techniques will show you how to stimulate your sexual energy. The exercises help strengthen the pelvic floor muscles, increase flexibility of the legs and pelvis, improve blood circulation to the uterus, and aid you in preparing for ritual intercourse.

Listed below are the seven exercises for energy and harmony, which gently activate the chakras, especially in the root and sacral centers (*muladhara* and *svadhisthana*, respectively), increasing body awareness as a whole. Activating the lower chakras is important because they optimize the vital power that affects sexuality. For example, your genitals will be provided with energy and potency. Fecundity will be enhanced, and the intensity of orgasm will be increased.

Ultimately, the exercises support the stomach and pelvic area and reinforce the quality of physical, mental, and spiritual pleasure.

In order to fully develop your sexual power, routinely practice Tantra-Yoga exercises. This will help establish a connection between head and pelvic region, a conjunction that is necessary to better engage your sexual energy. You can also intensify the effectiveness of the exercises if you observe the following recommendations.

Tips: How to Activate the Lower Chakras

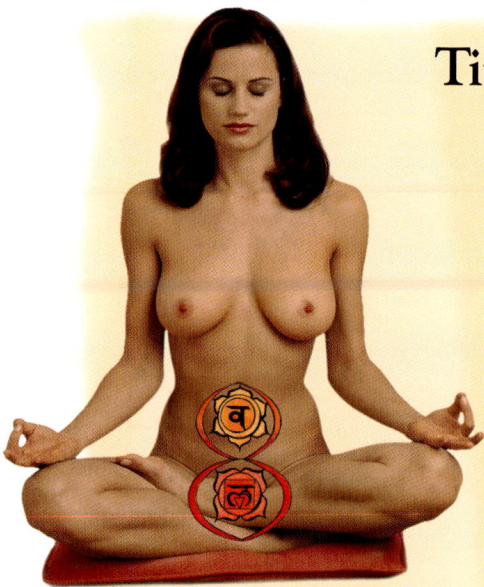

- Make sure you have sufficient range of motion. In order to become active, attempt moderate sports on a regular basis. If that doesn't appeal to you, try to take long walks every day.
- Always take time to go out and enjoy nature and cultivate your connection to the earth. As often as possible, walk barefoot, enjoy the air, and sunbathe (in moderation, of course, and with adequate sunscreen).
- Become intimate with your body. Massage yourself or let yourself be massaged, dance, play drums, or enjoy your body in a tender and erotic partnership.
- Wear comfortable, breathable clothing made from natural fibers—clothing you feel good wearing. Red and orange tones activate the lower chakras (see page 18), so buy clothes and decorate your bedroom with fabric, flowers, or rugs in these colors.
- Connect with elements of water to encourage your sacral chakra. Plan a holiday at the ocean or on a lake, swim regularly, enjoy a steam bath, or treat yourself at home to a hot bath and aromatic oils.
- Several essential oils have the ability to rouse the lower chakras, especially if you make sure to use only high-quality products. Pleasing scents to use are cloves, cypress, rosemary, sandalwood, bitter orange, and allspice. Put three to four drops of essence in an aroma lamp or a few drops mixed with milk in bathwater.
- Certain gemstones have the ability to carry energy to the lower chakras, making them

Tantra-Yoga Exercises

An important hint: the following Tantra-Yoga exercises are composed of different body positions, breathing techniques, and lessons in expanding your awareness. Even if they do not appear astounding at first, these specific exercises are very effective and you will feel the physical results in a very short time if you train with concentration. The exercises will strengthen the energy in the stomach and pelvic area and establish a good balance for the top-heaviness of our times; in other words, tiredness and

stronger and more forceful. Carry the stone in your pocket or directly against your skin. It can be a calming stone carried in your hand In order to waken the *muladhara* **(root) chakra, the following stones are suitable: ruby, red coral, spinel, sarder, red jasper, granite, or cat's eye. If you want to strengthen the** *svadhisthana* **(sacral) chakra, select tiger eye, gold topaz, jade, hyacinth, Fire opal, or sunstone.**

⑤ **Maintain your conscious awareness. This doesn't mean that should become an ascetic— Tantra rejects joylessness. Be free to enjoy the occasional glass of wine or piece of chocolate, but refrain from excess. Enjoyment has nothing to do with consuming. In general, do not overeat, and nourish yourself with fruits, vegetables, salad, milk, and wholegrain products.**

exhaustion from present-day life will fade, replaced by the awakening of new energies and bodily awareness. But be careful: if energies are activated too rapidly or have not been used in several years, unwanted results such as hot flashes, insomnia, or nervousness can occur. Simply put, if you train in the wrong way or begin Tantra-Yoga unprepared, you will experience negative results. It is not without reason that techniques that have the power to awaken kundalini, have been kept secret for hundreds of years!

Waking Concealed Energies

Traditionally, masters only imparted Tantra-Yoga exercises to students already trained in Yoga and consciousness-raising who were capable of assimilating these advanced techniques. This suggests that you should also prepare a foundation of training so the activated energies do not have an undesired outcome.

Therefore, before you perform exercises that awaken kundalini and the ensuing sexual energies, it is imperative that you gain some experience with the seven exercises for harmony and energy (see page 23). This will help you to cleanse and fortify your entire system, giving you the ability to do the exercises.

⑤ Perform the following tech-

Aromatic oils such as sandalwood or cloves help to awaken your lower chakras.

niques only once a day.

⑤ While exercising, remain tranquil and feel the inner you.

⑤ It is enough to begin a short program at first, selecting only a few exercises to start with. At first, pay more attention to those exercises that relax the pelvic muscles.

⑤ Always follow the exercises in the order given.

⑤ Always finish your personal program with a short meditation.

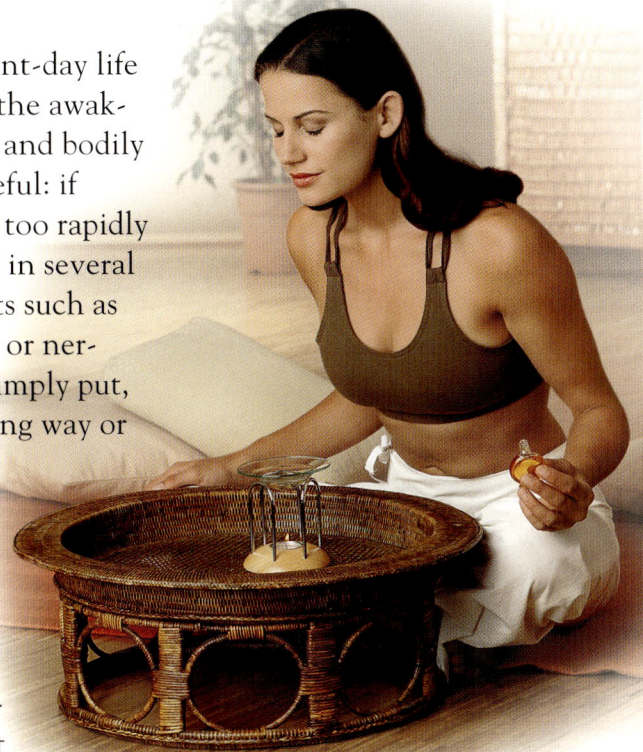

Getting Ready

1 Sit on your heels, either cross-legged or in a half-lotus position (see box at right). Keep your spine straight but allow your shoulder, neck, and facial muscles to remain relaxed. Place your hands on your knees with the palms facing up and form a ring with your index finger and thumb, a position that boosts concentration. Close your eyes and focus on your breathing. Inhale deeply through your nose and as you exhale, quietly repeat the mantra LAM (pronounced "long") seven times. This will activate the *muladhara* (root) chakra. Inhale deeply again through your nose and let the syllable LAM resound seven times in your head. Repeat the process three times while simultaneously concentrating on your coccyx and perineum, the region between your anus and outer genitals.

Inhale once again through your nose and say the mantra VAM as you exhale. This will activate the *svadhisthana* (sacral) chakra. As before, let the syllable resound in your head seven times as you focus on the area above the pubic bone, approximately a hand width below the navel.

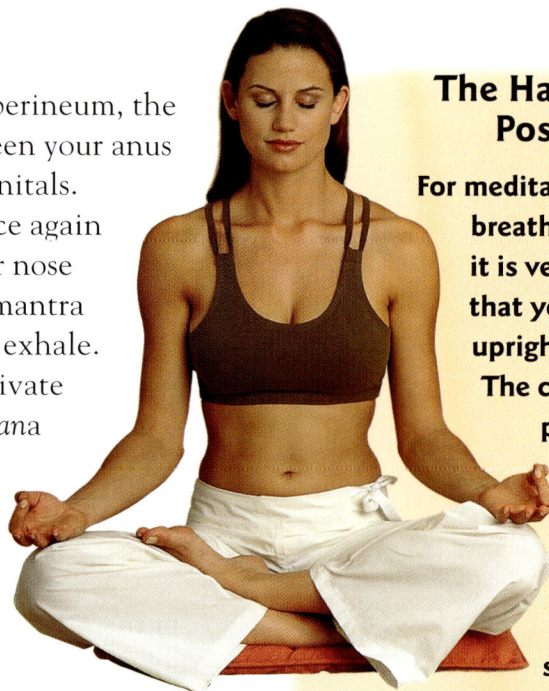

The Half-Lotus Position

For meditation and breathing purposes, it is very important that you sit solidly upright on the floor. The crossed-leg position is quite simple, but you may be much more comfortable if you place a small pillow under your backside.

For the half-lotus position, begin by angling your right leg so that you can pull your right foot as close to your body as possible. Next, angle the left leg and place the foot on your right thigh. Be a little patient if at first you do not feel comfortable in this position; you will soon master it if you practice conscientiously.

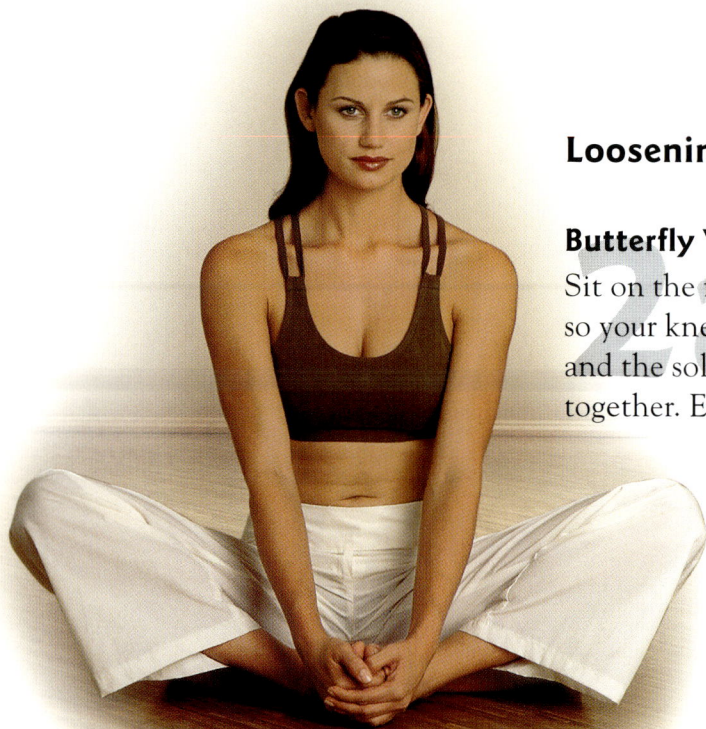

Loosening the Hips

Butterfly Wings

2a Sit on the floor. Angle your legs so your knees point to the sides and the soles of your feet are together. Enclose your feet with your hands and pull your heels as close to your body as possible; then move your knees alternately up and down, as you would move the wings of a butterfly. Perform this movement very gently and avoid any strain or painful effort.

Repeat this exercise again once or twice more, stretching your legs in between repetitions. The goal is to stretch the muscles of your hips, groin, and legs.

In this exercise, your legs move like butterfly wings, gently up and down.

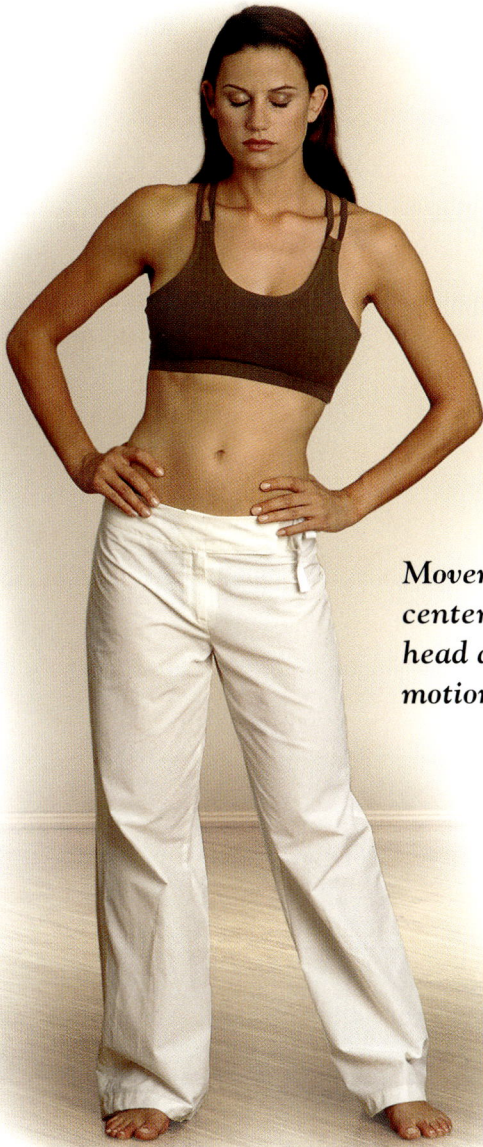

Pelvic Rotation

Stand straight with your feet about shoulder width apart and toes pointed forward. With hands on hips, begin rotating your pelvis; begin with smaller rotations that gradually become larger circles as you progress. Focus on your pelvis and genitals and pay attention to your movements—you want your head to stay still while your hips move. Perform this exercise first in clockwise, then counter-clockwise motion. Return to your starting position when finished.

Movement should stem from the center of the body while your head and torso remain as motionless as possible.

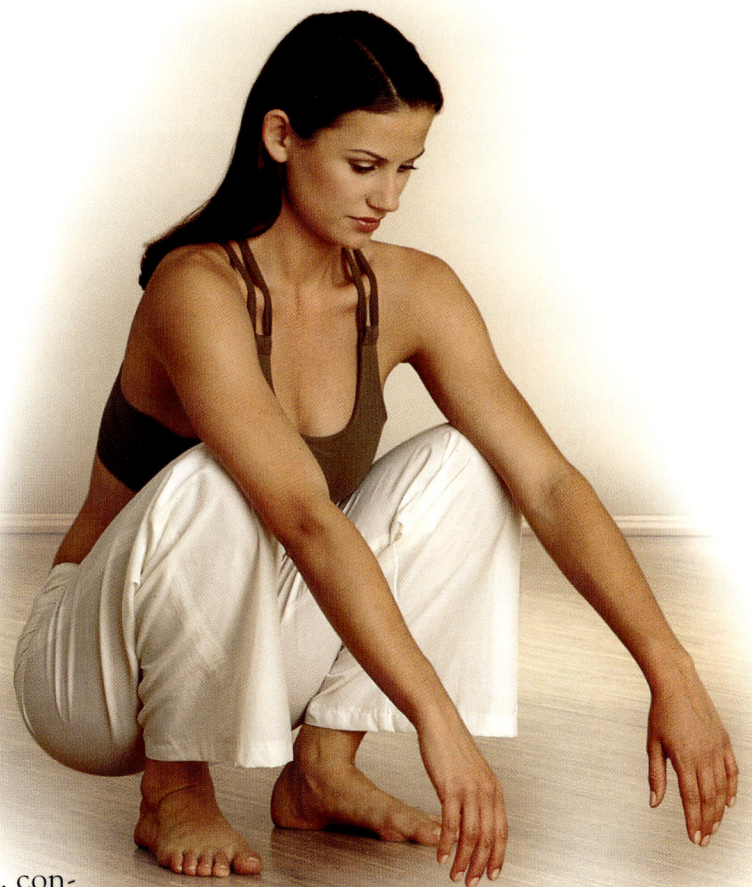

Low Crouch

Place your feet shoulder width apart and the toes pointed slightly outward. Slowly crouch down as far as you can. When you first begin, it is acceptable if your backside only reaches the level of your knees. Keep your spine as straight as possible and extend your neck muscles so you are looking down toward your lap. Place your upper arms on your knees and remember to keep the soles of your feet solidly on the floor. Breathe deeply seven times, constricting the pelvic floor muscles slightly upward each time you inhale, and relaxing them when you exhale. Slowly return to a standing position.

This exercise also strengthens your sense of balance.

Breathing Exercises

3 Through the following breathing techniques, you are able to recharge yourself with prana, the energy of life that courses throughout your entire body. Breathing awareness is important because it helps you establish a connection to the inner perceptions of your body and intensify them. Attention to these perceptions is important; it expands your ability to awaken the inner beloved.

The following exercises are known in Tantra as pranayama (control of energy and breath), and they are especially important in awakening the energy of kundalini. Always perform these exercises carefully and listen to what your body is saying—less is sometimes more!

Yoga Complete Breathing

3a In Tantra, the use of slow, deep breathing has a dual purpose— to raise the level of prana and to prolong orgasm, which increases sexual desire. Yoga complete breathing is a combination of stomach, side, and chest breathing patterns that are performed in a cross-legged or half-lotus position (see box on page 30).

When you first begin, use your hands to help you become aware of the different areas of breath; place one hand on your abdomen and the other on your chest while you inhale fully. Take the air first into your abdomen, which should noticeably expand outward. It should be drawn sideways into your sides so the ribs expand, and then into the chest. During this inhalation, a wavelike movement should develop from the bottom of your body and move upward.

When you finish inhaling, exhale as deeply as possible so your lungs are completely clear. Begin by inhaling and exhaling for eight seconds each. Later you will be able to inhale and exhale up to the count of sixteen. Repeat this technique at least five times.

Concentrate on how the breath flows throughout your body.

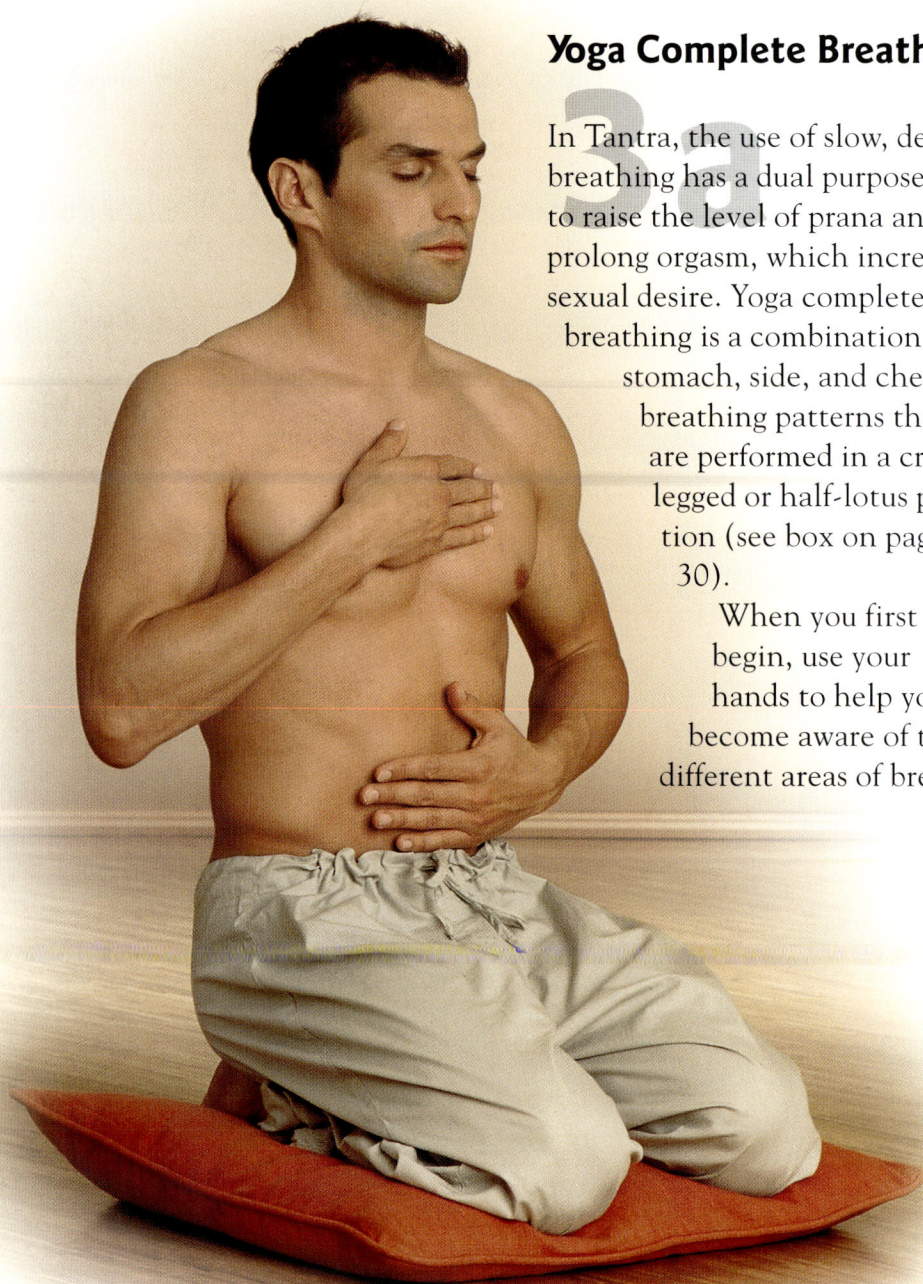

Bringing Shiva and Shakti into Harmony

3b

This breathing technique, also known as changing breath, brings Shiva and Shakti into harmony. The exercise balances the flow of energy in the main channels of the astral bodies, opens blocks and, most importantly, harmonizes both sides of the brain. Both male and female energies need to be in balance if a state of intense tranquility is to be achieved.

While sitting, inhale deeply through your nose. Press your right nostril gently closed with your thumb and exhale for eight seconds through the left one. Inhale again through the left nostril to another count of eight, then press it closed with your index finger, and exhale through the right. Repeat the pattern—left out, left in, right out, right in—several times while remaining as quiet and steady as possible.

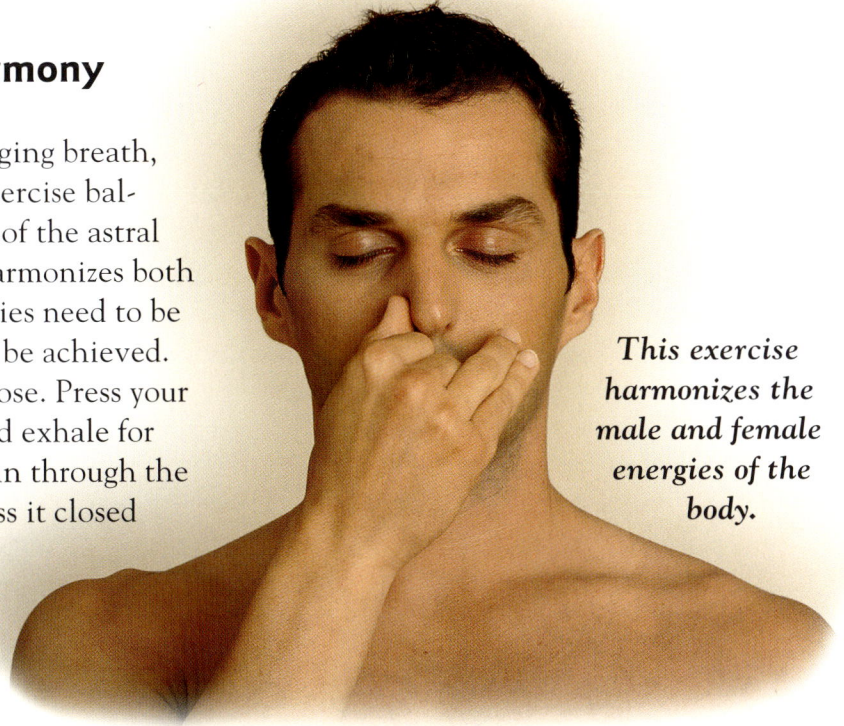

This exercise harmonizes the male and female energies of the body.

Prana—The Cosmic Life Energy

Only those who learn to master life energy will be able to experience the complete spiritual dimension of Tantra. A tantrician is aware that energy must be budgeted in order to store it in the chakras.

This energy is called prana, which describes the elementary power of all phenomena or the cosmic energy of life, which stimulates the body, soul, and spirit. Human beings are always surrounded by prana, which is visible in nature as light, heat, magnetism, and electricity, yet it cannot be experienced by those who are untrained in using this energy productively.

Our bodies are physiologically restored through prana by means of heat, light, and breathing, but Tantra requires additional mental stimulation of these energies in order to gain conscious awareness. Therefore, exercises like complete breathing and pranayama techniques are required in order to make prana more accessible to those who would utilize it as a precise energy. Those who have a high amount of prana available are usually mentally balanced, physically fit, and maintain high energy.

The best ways to accumulate prana are to:

🖰 Perform breathing and Tantra-Yoga exercises

🖰 Get sufficient sleep

🖰 Do moderate exercise on a daily basis

🖰 Meditate

🖰 Train your concentration

🖰 Develop all levels of your personality

🖰 Avoid frequent ejaculation

🖰 Enjoy life and live consciously

Prana is primarily wasted through:

🖰 An excess of alcohol and nicotine

🖰 Unhealthy, fatty foods with little vitamin content

🖰 Stress factors such as immoderate ambition, competitive sports, anxiety, or sorrow

🖰 Drugs

🖰 Mass media, pornography, addiction to luxury, or other vicarious pleasures

🖰 Lack of sleep and living against natural rhythms

🖰 Diversion, disorientation, aimlessness, and senselessness

Awakening Kundalini

There lies in each individual a tremendous amount of hidden potential. In Tantra, this is symbolized by kundalini, the coiled snake that sleeps at the base of the spine, waiting to be awakened. The purpose of the exercises introduced here is to arouse the power of kundalini in order to transform sexuality. Whether alone or exercising with a partner, they can be very effective.

Warming Kundalini

Stand straight with your legs slightly parted. Place the palm of your left hand on your abdomen approximately three fingers below your belly button, the right hand simply covering the left. Direct contact with the skin is very important so have your stomach completely uncovered before doing this exercise. Begin to breathe deeply, feeling the rise and fall of your abdomen with each intake of breath. Now close your eyes, feel how the floor bears your weight, and concentrate on your abdomen. With your hands, start making circular motions over your stomach: large circles at first, then concentric smaller ones at a faster pace so that the circular massage warms the skin. Perform the circles both clockwise and counter-clockwise. When you are finished, rest your hands in the same starting position, right hand over left.

Maintain a steady position for this exercise.

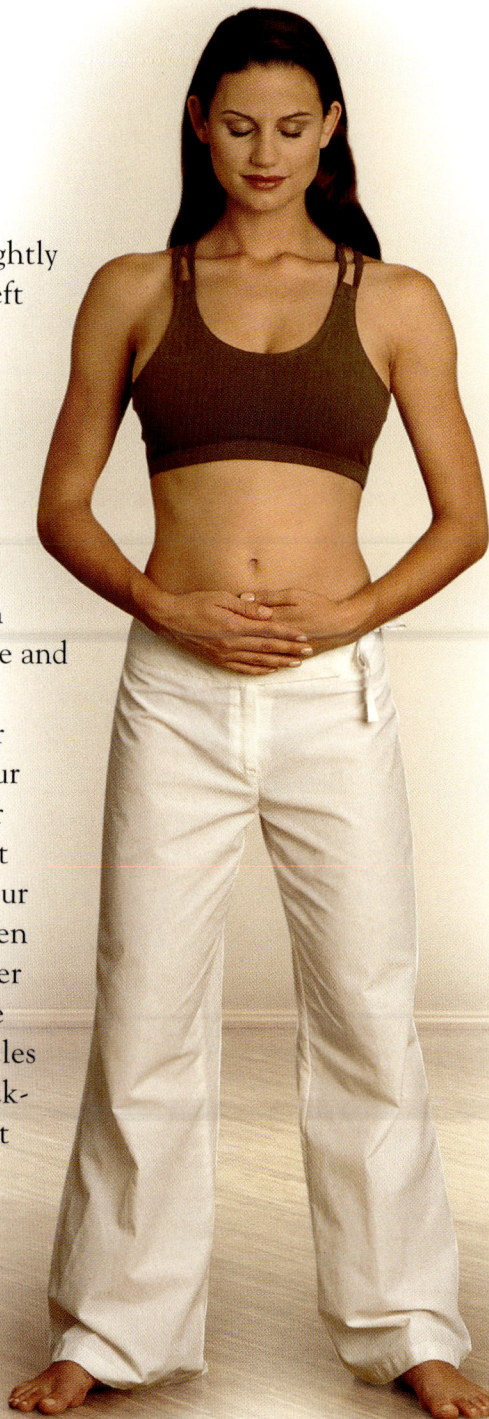

Letting Kundalini Rise

Sit in a cross-legged or half-lotus position (see box on page 30). Close your eyes and allow yourself to breathe freely. Concentrate on the moment and empty your head of all extraneous thoughts as you exhale deeply, bringing yourself into a completely relaxed state. Next, breathe through your nose eight times. At the last intake of breath, press your chin onto your chest and tense your stomach muscles by lifting them upward and in while you simultaneously tighten your sphincter. (These three actions of chin, stomach, and sphincter are called *bandhas*. Their purpose is to store prana and awaken energy).

   Hold your breath for eight seconds (*kumbhaka*) while you maintain the constriction of your chin (*jalandhara bandha*), your stomach (*uddiyana bandha*), and sphincter (*mula bandha*). During these eight seconds, imagine that a warm light from the lower chakra is rising up along your spine toward your navel. When it reaches that point, loosen your chin, stomach, and sphincter and exhale slowly through your nose.

During the first few weeks of exercise, this technique should be performed three times daily, with a later goal of ten times. Guide the harmonizing energies from the *muladhara* (root) chakra only toward your navel for the moment, but as you become more experienced, direct it toward the heart chakra, located in the middle of the chest.

The kundalini exercises consist of four phases:

🌀 Inhale for eight seconds.
🌀 Hold your breath for another eight seconds and constrict the three bandha openings while imagining the ray of light rising in your body.
🌀 Open the three areas and exhale slowly.
🌀 Breathe easily two or three times before repeating the exercise.

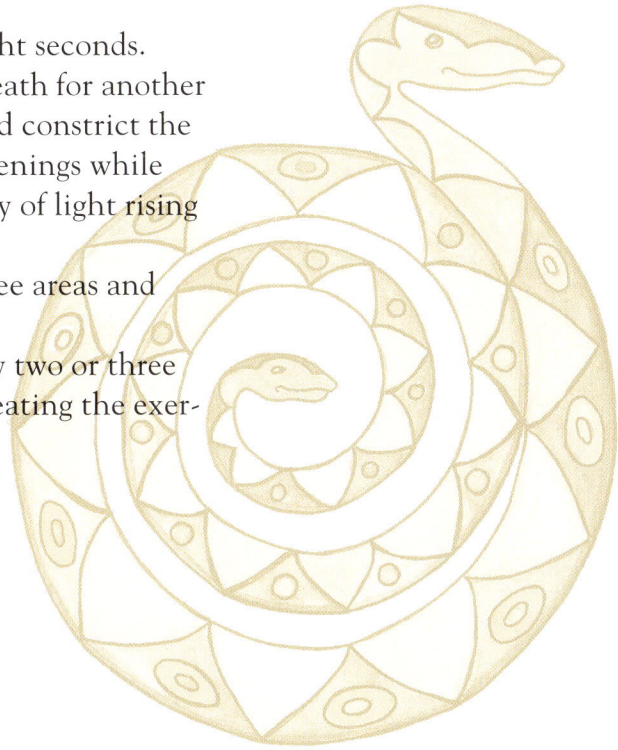

Conclusion

The following relaxation technique can be performed independently of your exercise regimen, in order to harmonize sexual power and supply your genitals with healing energy.

Lie on your back, close your eyes, and thoroughly relax all the muscles in your body. Place one hand on the center of your abdomen below the navel and the other hand on the pubic mound, directly above the genitals. Feel the rhythm of your breathing. As you inhale, consciously collect prana and direct the flow of energy into your chakras. Imagine this cosmic energy as a bright reddish ball of light that is exuding warmth as it flows from your hands into your lower body, filling your genitals with a pleasant sensation of heat. Breathe rhythmically for seven seconds as you maintain this visualization. Then, slowly place your hands on the floor. Remain in this position as you experience the effects of this exercise.

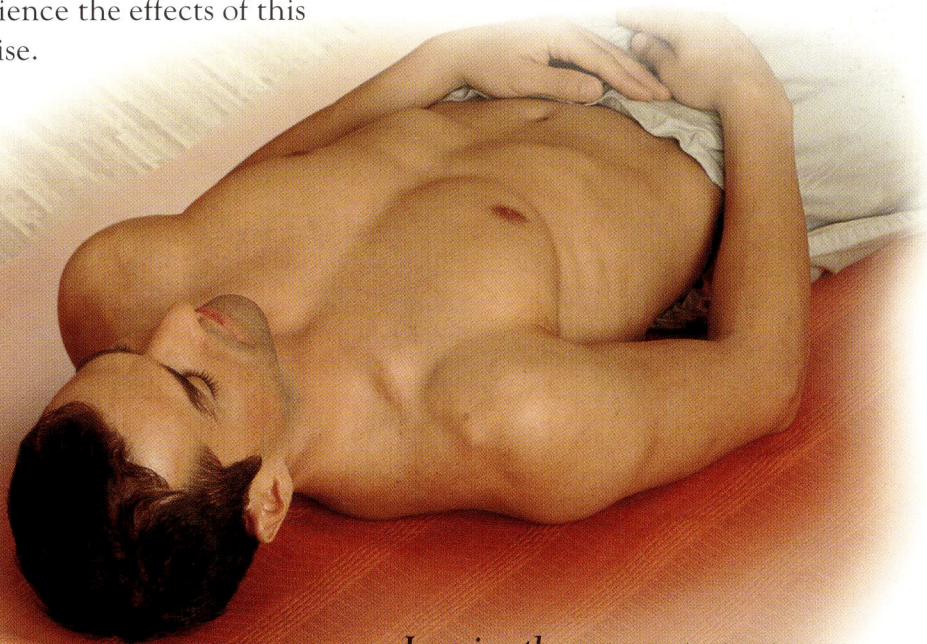

Imagine the energy as a warm, pleasant, and healing light.

Love Yourself

Developing a comfortable and loving attitude about yourself is an important step in Tantra. A successful relationship with a partner is only possible if you maintain a good relationship with yourself first.

In order to practice Tantra, you need to have a positive opinion of yourself because Tantra has nothing to do with external attributes. It is not about an ideal of beauty or the ability to perform acrobatic positions in bed. You do not have to be blessed with exceptional potency or penis length, nor do you have to be young and beautiful. Actually, quite the contrary: masters of Indian Tantra were seldom young and had no exceptional attributes. It is more important to accept your partner on a spiritual level and achieve the highest feelings of love, experience, and personal maturity than to focus on superficialities. Therefore, when you set out to discover your inner god or goddess through exploration of tantric secrets, you should search only inside yourself.

Games With Desire

The following games and exercises help you to acknowledge your body and sexuality. Their purpose is to help you discover yourself and your erotic side and to further develop sensitivity and openness. Open yourself up to your vital energies and throw all inhibition and taboos aside. Since the methods are sometimes very intimate, you should look for a private space where you can enjoy the time you need for yourself.

Before you can love someone, you must first like yourself.

Dancing Naked

Allow your energy to flow freely. Free yourself from inhibition: humans are naturally naked! Unfortunately, the influence of modern civilization has taught us to believe that nudity is unnatural and cause for shame. This sense of fear regarding your (naked) body or sexuality, or the sexuality of your partner, is a barrier to spiritual and ecstatic sex.

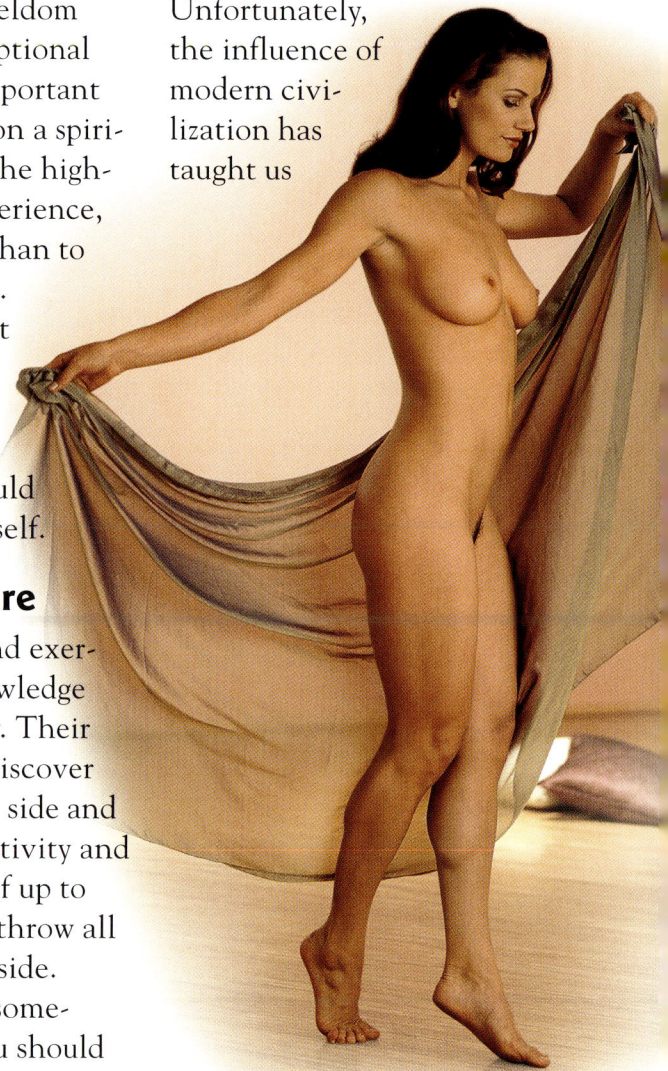

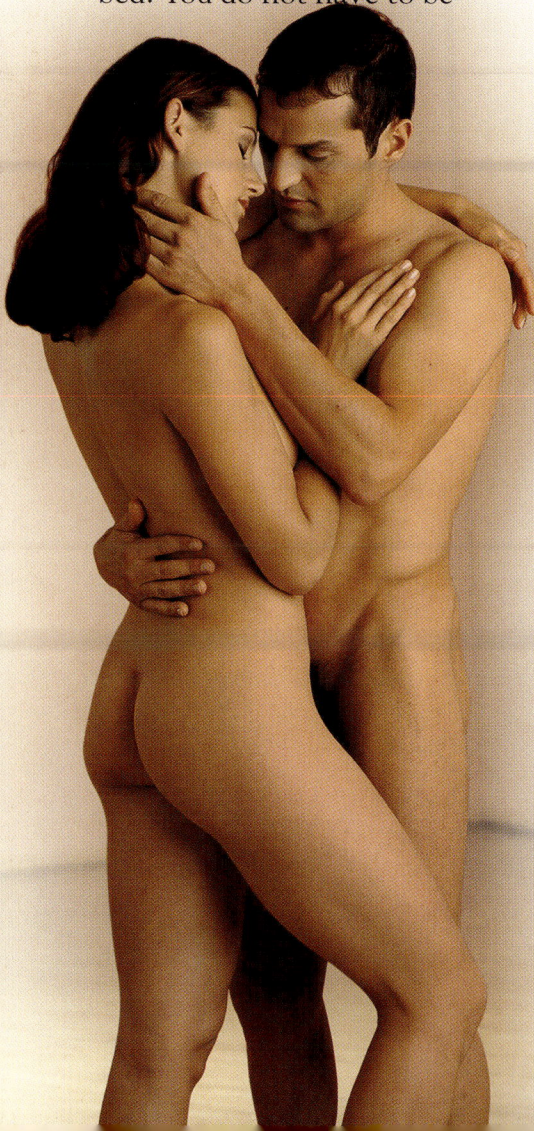

Free Yourself These obstacles can be easily overcome. For example, you can use every opportunity to liberate yourself from the confines of clothing. You can walk barefoot in the summer to absorb energy from the earth. Another good way to experience your body is to dance naked.

Select music that inspires you, such as rhythmic drum music or something slow and meditative. Let the music wash over you and flow through your body as you move. Do not merely use your legs, rather allow your entire body to glide and accompany you for as long as you choose. As you dance, remain consciously observant of your body—the manner in which you dance gives a lot of information about how you interact with your body and your sexuality.

Mirror Image

Even though you should also touch yourself when looking into a mirror, contact is less important here than your ability to consciously see yourself. Very few people take the time to examine their bodies closely, yet only those who consciously observe themselves with total concentration can be sensitively attuned to a partner.

When using a mirror, be sure it is a large one, preferably floor length and freestanding, and use soft lighting such as candles or red and yellow incandescent bulbs that illuminate the skin.

Sit cross-legged before the mirror and first observe your face. Look into your eyes for a time, and then concentrate on your lips, stroking them gently with your fingertips. Let your fingers glide down over your chin, throat, and breasts, continually caressing yourself as you gaze into the mirror. Now slowly stand up to examine your abdomen, thighs, and pubic area.

Loving Observation This is not a judgmental look in the mirror! Look at your abdomen, pubic area, and pelvis, and accept these pleasure-giving areas as parts of yourself. Gently caress them. Caress your hips and thighs, noticing how your hands pamper your lower body.

Turn around so your back faces the mirror: look over your shoulder and appreciatively consider your back and buttocks.

Now lie down on the floor directly in front of the mirror, preferably on a

Experience the uniqueness of your own body.

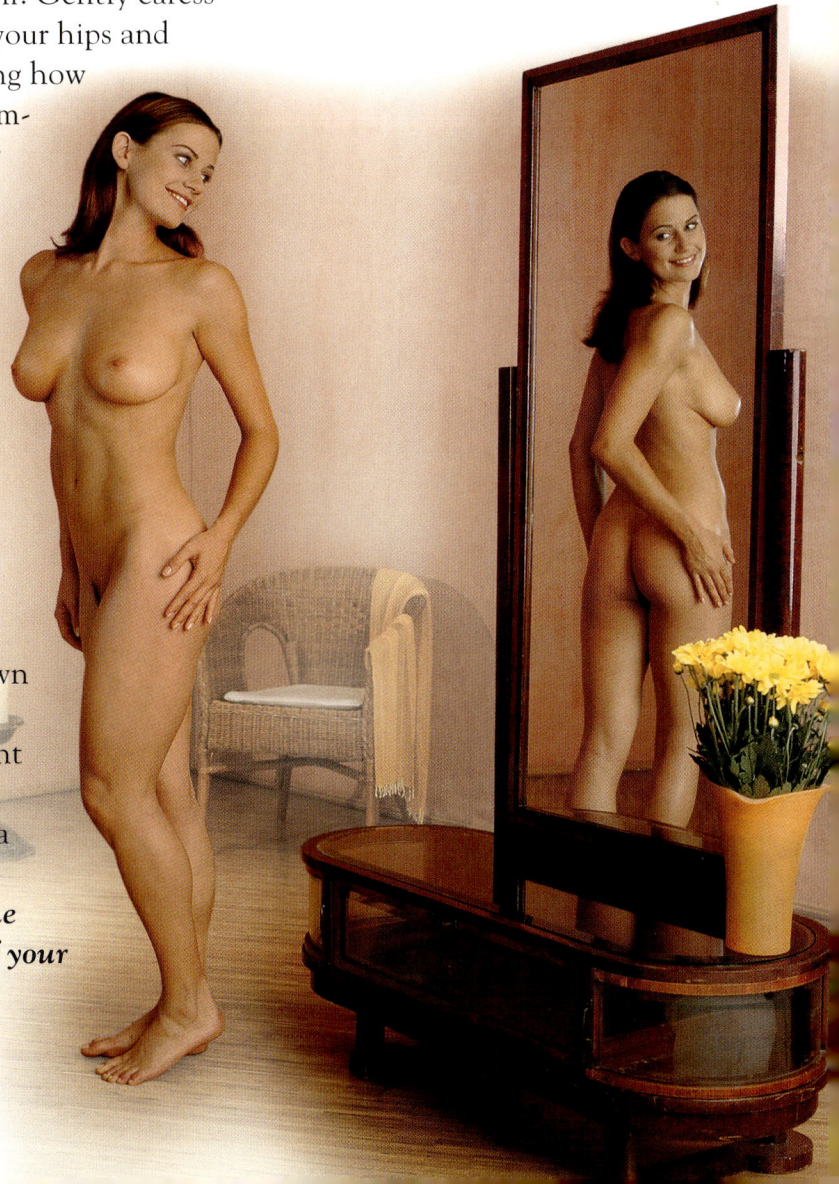

blanket and with a pillow raising your head. Open your legs and examine your outer genitals, the outer labia and the shape of your pubic mound.

Gently open your labia with your fingers and observe your labia minora, the clitoris, and vaginal entrance. If you are a man, observe the shape of your testicles and penis, gently pulling back the foreskin. Memorize your body and finish this exercise gradually.

Explore Yourself

As we have seen, there are many ways in which to discover your body and develop your erotic charisma—observing yourself in a mirror, dancing, going about naked, or caressing yourself.

Touching yourself is an important preliminary step toward intercourse with your partner, so do not shy away from stroking and exploring your own body thoroughly. The following suggestions should be explored in a playful and intuitive manner and can be adjusted to your needs.

Finding Your Own Ritual

Before beginning a ritual of self-exploration, you should take a shower, moisturize your body with lotion, and carefully wash your hands. Lie naked on your bed or on a blanket on the floor in a room warm enough for comfort. Lie on your back with your knees spread so the soles of your feet are against each other. Place your hands on the floor, close your eyes, and concentrate on the inside of your body. During this entire exercise, your eyes should remain closed and your breathing relaxed.

Touching Yourself In the first part of this exercise stroke yourself with your left hand and become attuned to your body. Imagine that your left hand is that of someone else, perhaps a lover caressing you. Adjust your mind-frame to "I am allowing myself to be touched."

Place your left hand on your left knee and begin stroking your thigh while imagining that it is someone else touching you. Take your time in visualizing this.

Slowly glide your hand upward and caress your hips, then turn your attention to your abdomen and breasts. Caress your skin very gently and massage these areas with circular movements.

Enclose your nipple between thumb and index finger, applying a little pressure as you rub back and forth. Breathe softly and continue to imagine that you are being touched by someone else's hand.

Eventually, bring your hand upward and caress your throat and face, gliding your fingers over lips, cheeks, and ears. Now let your hand wander from your face downward toward your genitals.

Variation for Women

Direct your attention to your pubic area and, with your left hand, explore the characteristics of your pubic mound. Run through your pubic hair and let your finger glide along the lips of your outer labia. Take the labia between two fingers and press gently while breathing deeply through your mouth.

Carefully pull apart your labia with two fingers and, with your middle finger, stroke along the inner skin of your labia and vaginal entrance.

Explore your body through gentle, loving caresses.

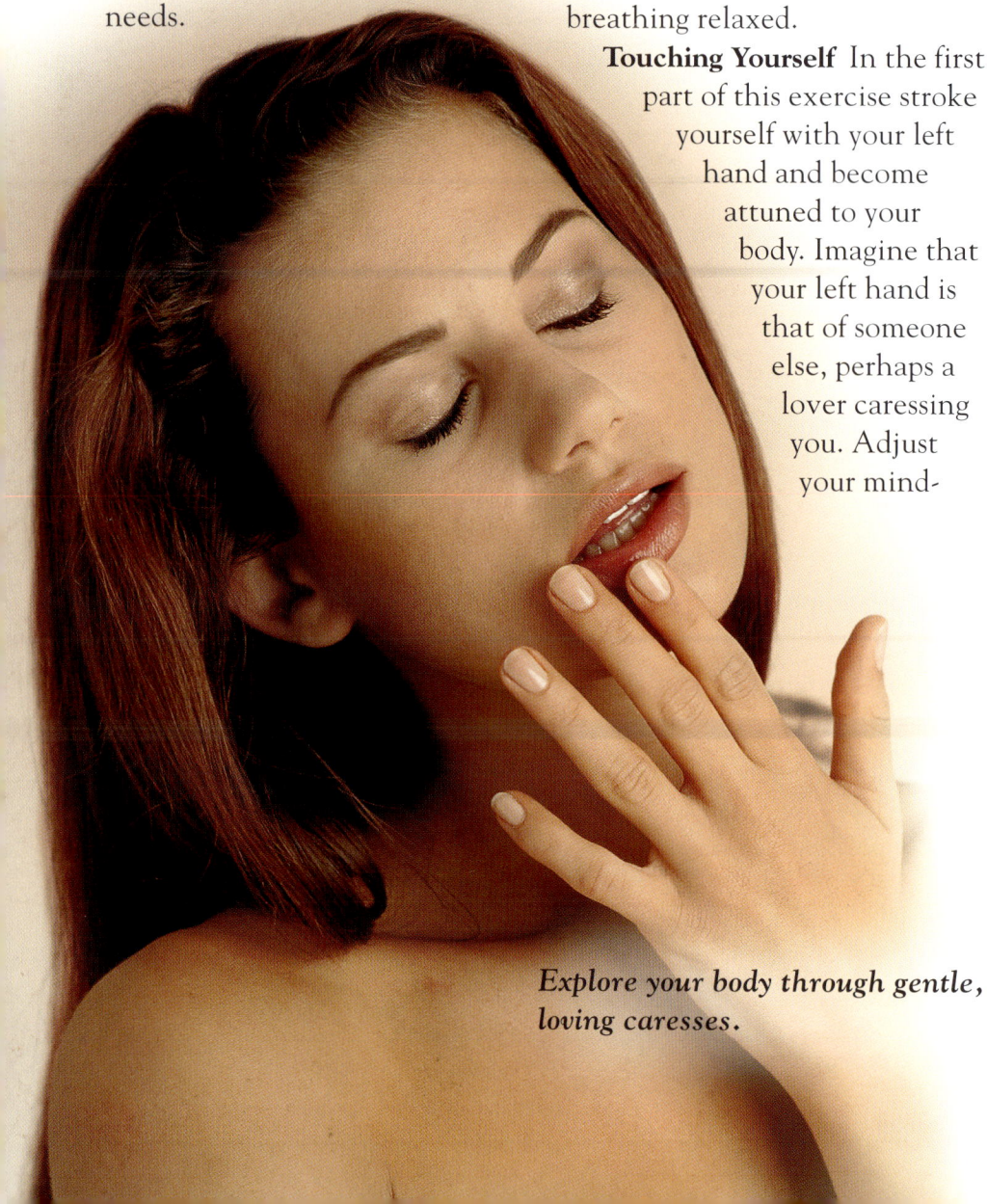

Vary the rhythm of your movements. Now explore the inside of your vagina by placing two moistened fingers inside and feeling along the walls, lingering on the areas which are especially sensitive. Tense your pelvic muscles and try to enclose your finger within your vagina as tightly as possible with your vaginal muscles. Continue to imagine that these fingers exploring the intimate regions of your body are those of someone else.

Now move your fingers out and place between your labia minora. With soft circular movements, begin to stroke your clitoris and observe the effect on your pleasure when you vary the movement or pressure. Remember to keep your focus on the sensations in your genitals, not

in your hand or fingers. Let your hand rest on your vulva, then finish this self-exploration ritual by putting your hands again on the floor and closing your legs.

Variations for Men

Direct your attention to your genitals by feeling the contours of your testicles. Gently stroke the sensitive skin of this region, moving along the perineum, located between the testicles and anus. Imagine that your hand is that of someone else, for example, a lover exploring your body.

Now place your left hand on your penis and glide up and down its length. Form a ring with your thumb and index finger and stroke upward until you reach the band of your foreskin (frenulum). Slowly caress the

underside of your penis, concentrating on the most sensitive areas, then once again forward until you reach the glans.

Now move the foreskin slowly up and down. At first, perform this movement with your thumb and index finger, then with the hand, which should enclose the entire penis below the glans.

Continue to imagine that it is a lover's hand moving up and down your penis. Vary the pressure and rhythm, breathe deeply, and feel the waves of ecstasy spread through your body. Finish this exercise without ejaculating! The goal of the self-exploration ritual is not masturbation, but the conscious perception of a "stranger's" hand, and the reaction caused in the body.

Male and Female Genitals

When performing the ritual of self-exploration, treat yourself lovingly and examine every single part of your genitals extensively.

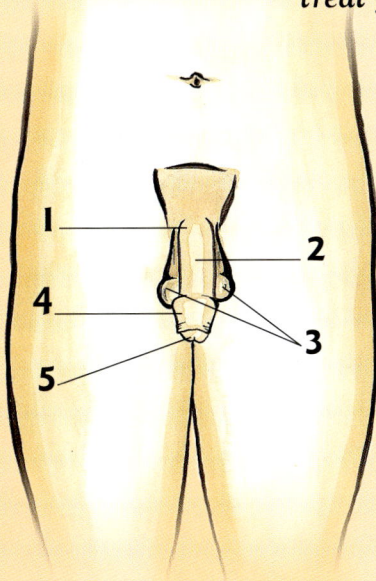

1 *Shaft of the penis*
2 *Penis*
3 *Testicles*
4 *Foreskin*
5 *Glans*

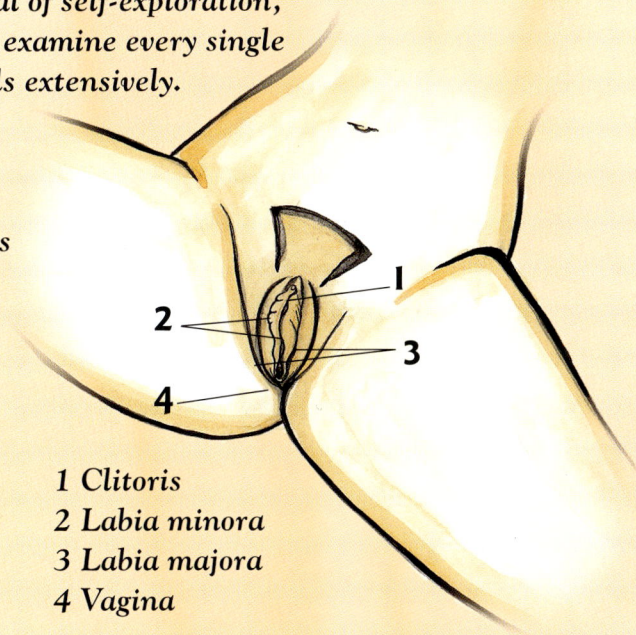

1 *Clitoris*
2 *Labia minora*
3 *Labia majora*
4 *Vagina*

Step Two of the Ritual

Take a short break between step one and step two of the self-exploration ritual. Walk around the room and shake your arms and legs, then lie down again on your back. Repeat all the steps described in step one, this time using your right hand to stroke yourself and focusing on the sensations in your hand instead of your body.

The purpose of step one was to imagine that someone else's hand was exploring your body; the goal is now to be conscious of what your hand feels when you are caressing the body of someone else. If you are able to achieve this alternate impression, you will see how large the difference in perception is.

As soon as you have finished step one, end this exercise by placing both hands on your lower abdomen. Become aware of the energy created by the ritual through sexual arousal and collected in the lower chakras; then imagine this energy slowly spreading throughout your entire body.

Sensuality in Daily Life

The ritual of self-exploration is a very intense exercise used to enhance body awareness, but it is also possible to develop this awareness in daily life and without ceremony. How? By using every possibility to consciously and lovingly touch yourself! Whether you are riding in a train, standing in a waiting room, or just comfortably sitting on your sofa, you can always place your hands on your abdomen or thighs and lightly massage yourself. At home, of course, you can touch

Touch yourself as gently as a lover would.

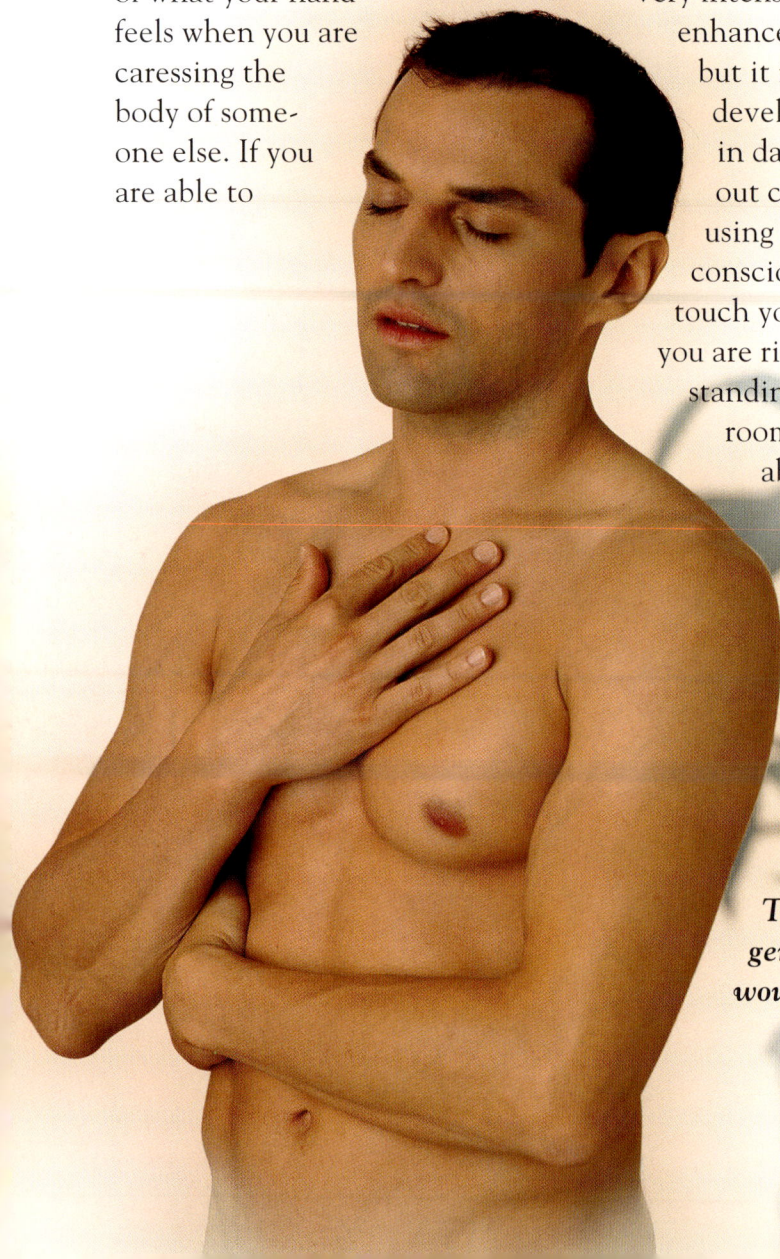

your pubic area and breasts. Just remember that it is important to train yourself in body awareness by always using both perspectives of the ritual—feel the shapes, warmth, and textures of the body through your hands while at the same time concentrating on the sensations in your body.

Indulge Yourself Enjoy sensuality in your daily life as much as possible. Treat yourself to long baths, go to a sauna, or moisturize yourself with scented creams. A self-massage also helps amplify pleasurable feelings within the body. Spread almond oil or special massage oils over your arms, legs, abdomen, hips, and chest and use circular movements to massage the oil into your skin. You'll feel good for some time afterward.

Training the Pelvic Floor

The following exercises help you recognize and strengthen the different muscles of the pelvic floor.

Control over the body is a must for every tantrician since intensifying sexual pleasure is only successful if you are completely familiar with your body and free of inhibitions. Exercises that strengthen the muscles used in intercourse are often considered unseemly, but they are the foundation on which you develop and expand your sexual energy. Techniques to control pelvic floor muscles have been cultivated for millennia in Tantra.

Muscles of the Pelvic Floor

The musculature of the pelvic floor resembles a figure eight and is comprised of the vagina or root of the penis in the upper region, and the bladder and rectum in the lower. Of particular importance is the musculus bulbocavernosus, which surrounds the genitals. In our society, strengthening these muscles is usually recommended only in connection with pregnancy or incontinence; the ability to use them to increase desire between yourself and your partner remains widely unknown.

Increasing Desire

An ancient Tantric text, the Ananga-Ranga, describes vaginal muscle control that is especially distinctive in some countries. For example, Abyssinian women could cause ejaculation through the mere flexing of their vaginal muscles while the rest of their body remained motionless. In southern India, young women still learn the art and can even imitate the opening and closing of a hand.

This is a basic technique of Tantra that is not only used to bring your partner to ecstasy, but to also intensify the female orgasm and desire for sexual intercourse.

Prolonged Erection Men have as much reason as women to train their pelvic floor muscles. The muscle, which encompasses the root of the penis, is what raises the penis in an upward motion; therefore, both the length and strength of an erection can be improved through regular training. The most important technique for training the genitals is *mula bandha*, which activates your vitality and sexual energy.

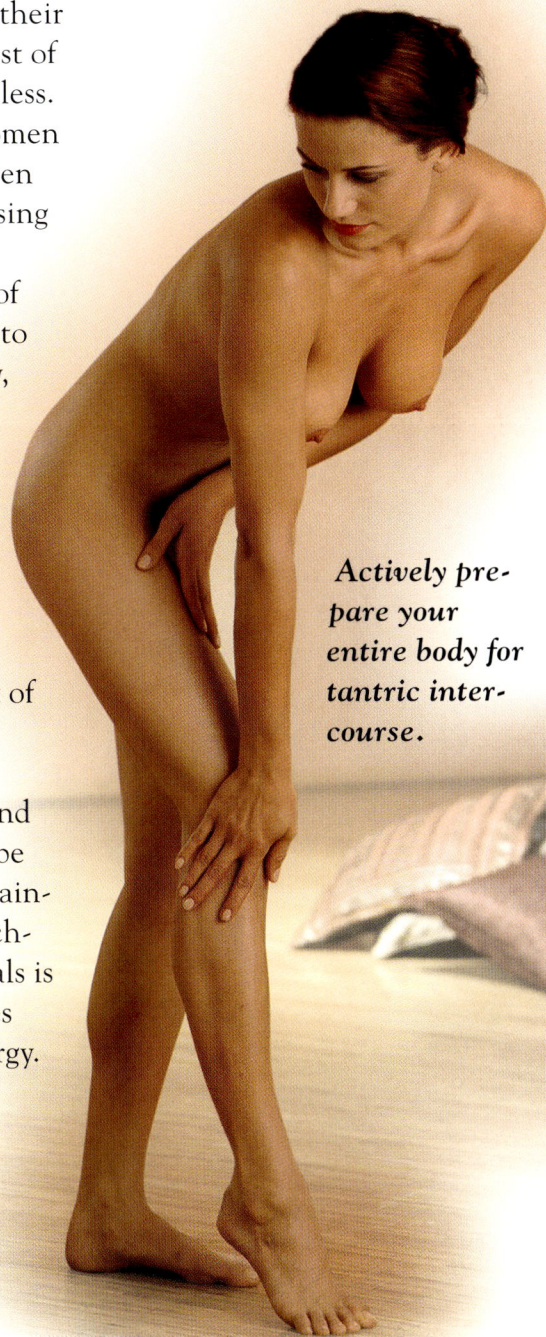

Actively prepare your entire body for tantric intercourse.

Mula Bandha

One of the most effective exercises to strengthen the pelvic floor is *mula bandha*.

Lie on the floor with your head relaxed against it and your thighs pulled toward your chest. Cross your legs in such a way that your right ankle is resting on top of the left. Putting your hands through the center of your open legs, grasp your left ankle with your right hand, and your right arch with your left. Lastly, put the tip of your tongue against your palate directly behind your incisors. In this position, you will close two important energy channels.

Now relax your arms, legs, face, and abdomen. Let your breath go in and out without any interference, and concentrate on the region of your rectum, perineum, and outer genitals. With each exhalation, direct energy to these areas.

Step One

Now begins the most important part of the exercise. As you inhale, press your sphincter muscles slightly outward. While exhaling, tense the entire pelvic floor musculature and contract your sphincter muscles. Females should spread the contraction forward from the anus until a distinct twitch is felt in the labia; males should spread the contraction from the anus until a distinct pull is felt on the testicles. Then release the pelvic contraction and breathe fully. Repeat this process of muscle tension and relaxation at least seven times, then relax by uncrossing your legs and lying flat on your back. *Mula bandha*, also known as the mare exercise, should be performed twice a day, either in the morning or evening.

Step Two

The second step of *mula bandha* is a refinement of the first. This next exercise is a very intimate one, but there is no better technique available to differentiate between the muscles of the anus

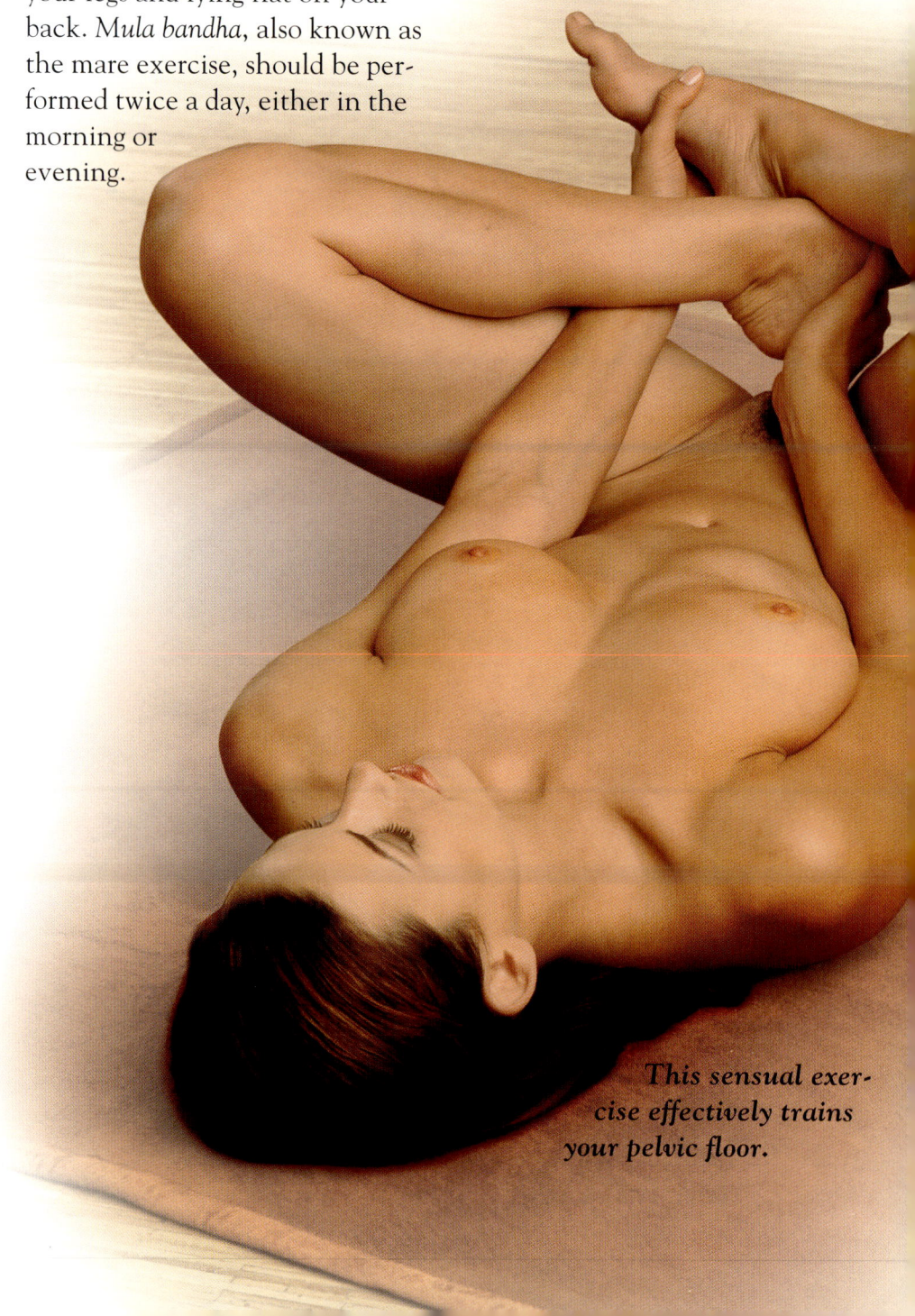

This sensual exercise effectively trains your pelvic floor.

and those of the vagina or the root of the penis.

If you can channel your concentration to your genital musculature, you will have the ability to not only intensify your orgasms, but also to control them, which is important for men who ejaculate too quickly. **Feeling the Pelvic Floor** Before you begin this exercise, be sure to empty your bladder and your bowels and wash your hands thoroughly. You will need lubricating jelly for this exercise.

Lie on your back and spread your legs apart. Women should then guide a finger of the left hand into the vagina and one from the right hand—covered with lubricating jelly—into the anus. Slide the fingers in slowly and carefully. Men should do this exercise by first placing their left hand on the shaft of the penis so that the middle finger touches the perineum and the palm is on the underside of the penis. The activity of the musculature is more prevalent if the penis is only half erect. Next slide a finger of the right hand—covered with lubricating jelly—into the anus.

Now concentrate on the region of the pelvic floor, genitals, and anus. Tense your muscles so they tightly constrict around your finger, then add more pressure. Men will feel

their penis lift and contract while women will feel their finger become enclosed within their vaginal muscles. Repeat the tension and relaxation sequence several times and vary the rhythm of the movement.

Differentiate Between the Muscles

Now attempt to apply tension to the sphincter only. This will require some practice, but it is more a matter of concentration than will. While the finger in the anus should be tightly enclosed within the muscles, women should only feel a slight pressure of the vaginal muscles. Men should notice that when the sphincter is truly contracted, the penis lifts as little as possible.

Now try this exercise the opposite way: the sphincter should receive minimal tension while the vaginal or penile musculature is constricted as tightly as possible.

As you continue to practice this exercise, you will be able to tighten the muscles independently of each other. During sexual intercourse, faster tension/relaxation sequences will stimulate orgasmic reaction and intensify feelings of desire.

Mula Bandha During Intercourse

Naturally it is important to try this technique during intercourse with your partner. While engaging in sex, keep your body absolutely motionless and only communicate through the contractions of your vaginal or penile musculature. Feel how your partner's muscles constrict then respond with rhythmical tension and relaxation of your pelvic floor. Alternate your movements, and experience how your awareness toward your body's sexual reactions become more refined over time.

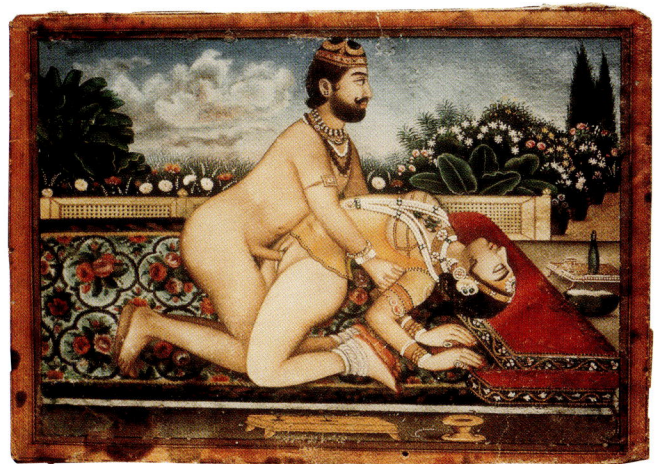

Regular training of Mula Bandha strengthens the pelvic floor muscles and intensifies the sexual sensation of both partners.

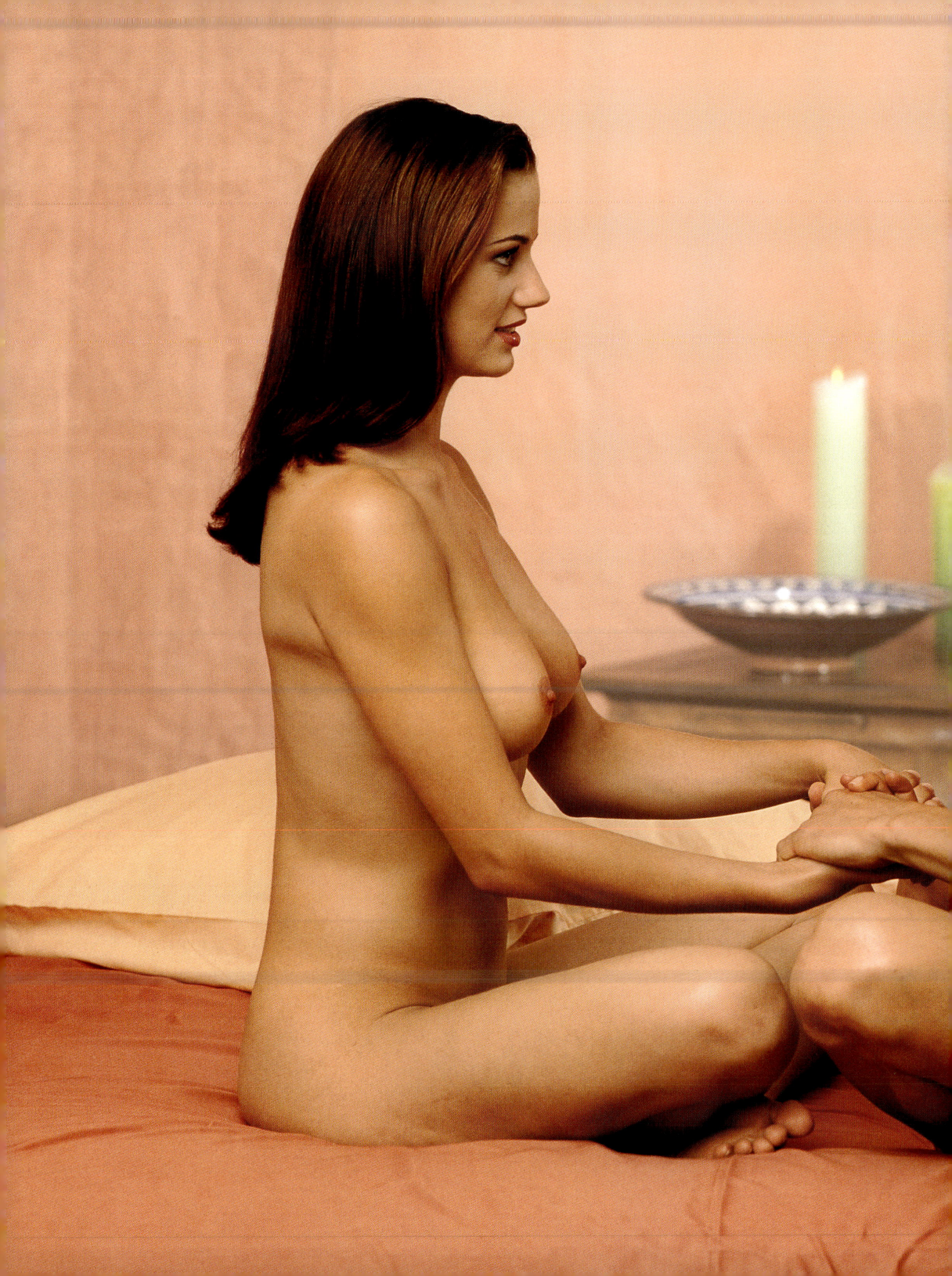

Time for Sensuality

Aesthetics, beauty, and sensuality are at the center of every tantric encounter. The many intimate rituals and erotic games entice you into the world of intense sensory experience. Colors, smells, and sounds help revitalize the game of love. Fervent embraces, pleasant caresses, and tender massages not only awaken fantasy; they break through the established pattern of relationships and introduce possibilities for a new, sensitive interaction.

Tantra Rituals

Now that you are familiar with some techniques that strengthen your sexual energy and heighten the awareness you have of your body, it's time for you and your partner to plunge into the world of sensory experience.

The following suggestions are used to prepare Shiva and Shakti for the different positions of Tantra. All these erotic games, exercises in energy exchange, and sensual massage, can also be performed independently of the *maithuna* ritual, or exercises that prepare you for sexual intercourse.

The exercises help you to:
- Awaken all your senses
- Promote desire and arousal in both partners
- Breathe new life into a stagnant relationship
- Discover the playful side of sexuality
- Exchange male and female energy
- Communicate in a mental-sensual manner
- Develop trust in and understanding of one another

As with most tantric exercises, those for sensuality require that you remain creative, spontaneous, and open-minded. Follow your childlike curiosity and be willing to experiment! Be attentive to the needs of both yourself and your partner and remember that these suggestions are not rules; they are merely a guide toward better understanding and compatibility between two people who want to enrich their shared experience.

Inner and Outer Moods

Tantra differs from ordinary sexual intercourse through its

Rituals and erotic games help you and your partner become closer to each other.

spiritual dimension, series of rituals, conscious awareness, and most importantly, the atmosphere where intercourse takes place; therefore aesthetics, beauty, self-assurance, and sensory perception play a large role. It is irrelevant whether you and your partner prepare for tantric intercourse through the *maithuna* ritual or by enjoying erotic massage. What is of utmost importance is that you maintain the right frame of mind. Always practice tantric exercises with the attitude, "As you make your bed, so you lie in it."

Break Through Routine Having the right mood for the time you would like to share with your partner is the first and perhaps most important step toward a sensual-spiritual encounter. To accomplish this, you must transform the surroundings of your love nest as well as yourself in order to break the daily routine.

Become Attentive Tantra is above all an engagement of conscious awareness. You will only be able to experience the secrets of these love arts in their entirety if you refine your sensory perception and train your cognitive skills. It is not always easy to concentrate on these skills when one is untrained in sexuality and works toward mere gratification.

Gratification is geared toward a sense of satisfaction rather than an

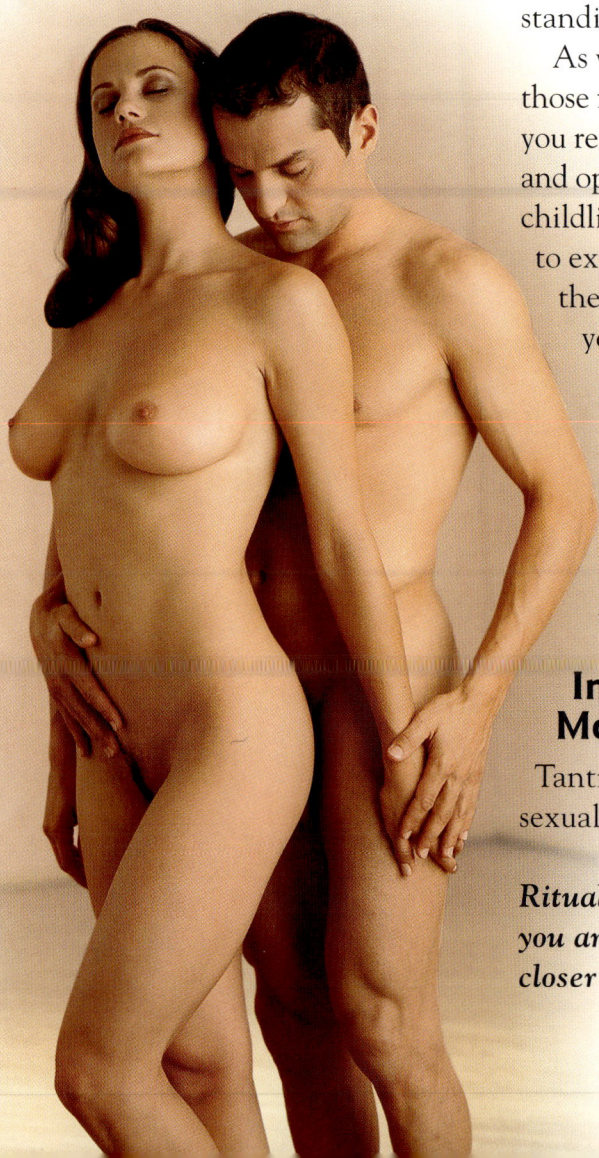

experience of sex as a holy action, but it still maintains a power that should not be underestimated. When one works to gratify, all processes are automatically driven, one is involved in one's own pleasure, and the partner is used as a tool to satisfy one's personal needs. **Developing Rituals** Tantra is not something that can be done quickly. It is a process that requires time and effort. Take the time to develop all the steps for a tantric encounter: greeting each other, transforming a room into a temple of desire, bathing together, sensual massage, and the culmination, sexual intercourse. All these steps are the rituals of Tantra.

Many people are skeptical when they hear the word "ritual." They assume it means something mysterious or even indecent, however most of us already perform rituals such as breakfast together on Sunday mornings, birthday parties, or holiday celebrations—any situation that we observe in a festive way. The rituals of Tantra help you find inner tranquility by discarding superficialities and allowing your thoughts to focus on the essentials.

Traditional Tantra Rituals

As far as we know, the traditional rituals of Tantra in ancient India usually lasted several days and required many years of intense preparation. They were also closely linked with Hindu culture and only performed under the supervision of a tantric master. Naturally, these same rituals would not be possible for modern people in the West, but the basic elements and principles behind them can be utilized by any open-minded couple. Have the courage to create your own ritual! You will find inspiration in the following section.

This eighteenth-century painting on wood portrays The Ode to the Joys of Physical Love.

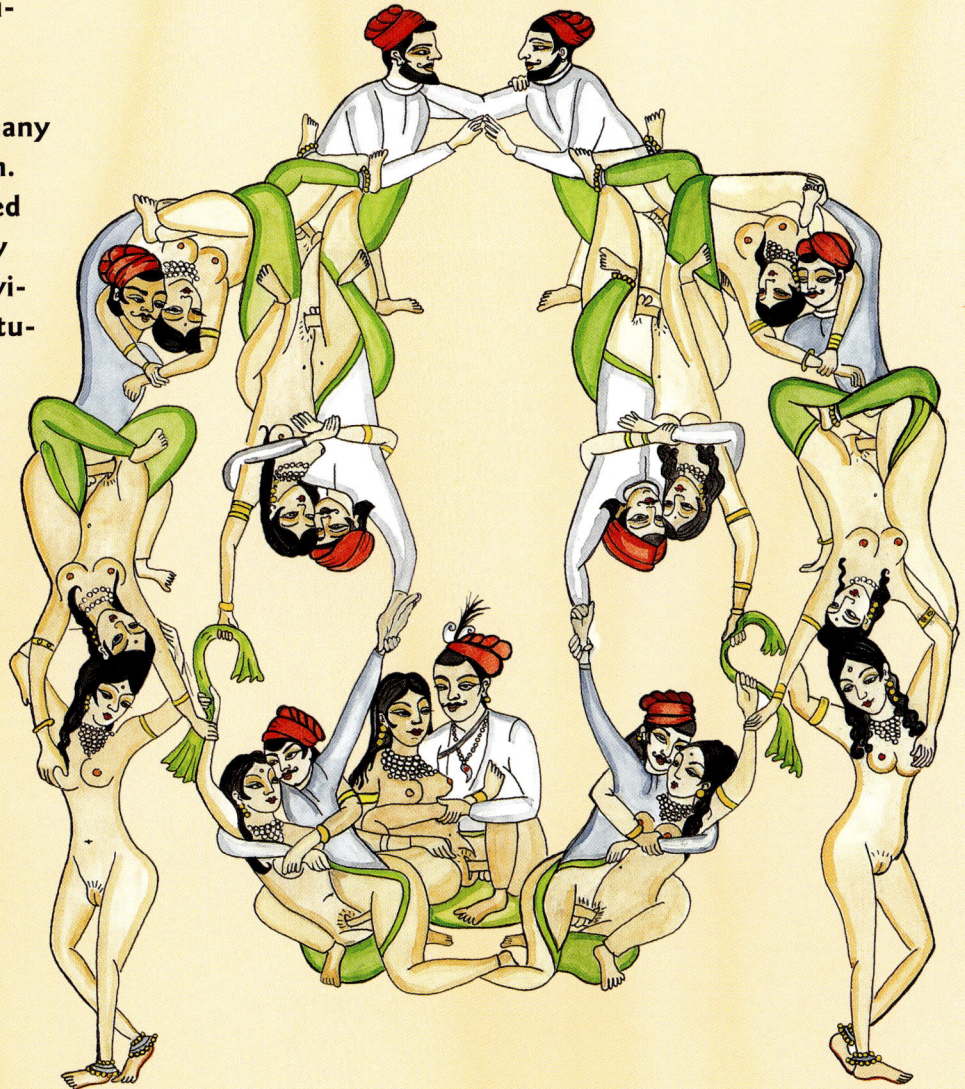

How to Evoke a Tantric Atmosphere

Using your imagination, transform a room in your house or apartment into a tantric playground. The only requirement is that you create a room in which you and your partner feel calm and comfortable.

Snuggle Warmly

It is important that your Tantra room have a comfortable temperature. If necessary, heat it thoroughly beforehand so it is possible to perform sensual foreplay as well as sexual intercourse totally naked. Also have soft blankets ready so that you may cover up and maintain body warmth as needed.

Be Undisturbed

In order to abandon yourself to uninhibited love-play, make absolutely sure that no one—roommates, children, pets, the postman—will disturb you. If need be, close the door and turn off the phone. Do whatever is necessary to ensure privacy for yourself and your lover.

You should also remove from your garden of desire objects such as the television, other electrical appliances, and shelves containing files and bills. The emptier the room, the easier it is to shut out distractions and concentrate totally on one another and your enjoyment.

The Manner of Love

For an intimate meeting, you will need an altar in your temple of love. It should consist of an appealing and comfortable rest area. You could make your bed the center of your tantric adventure, but this is recommended only if it is large enough (approximately two by two meters), and not so soft that exercises and positions become too difficult because you sink too deeply into the mattress.

In most cases, Indian followers of Tantra practice in open, grassy areas that they cushion with pillows and blankets. They believe that the fewer restrictions placed upon freedom of movement, the better the enjoyment.

There are many alternatives to a standard bed; for example, a large woolen carpet placed in the middle of the room is just as effective, especially if you cover it with a sheet and two or three soft blankets. Futons and other types of mattresses that sit directly on the floor are another possibility. Whatever your preference, always try to have many pillows, towels, and blankets nearby in order to make yourself genuinely comfortable.

Subdued Lighting

A further point to consider is appropriate lighting. When practicing Tantra or sensuous massage you must be able to see your partner. For a tantrician, sex in the dark is inconceivable since looking into the eyes of a lover is an important component of tantric intercourse. This doesn't mean that the room should be inundated with glaring light; on the contrary, the lighting should be soft and restful. An open fireplace would be ideal since it provides light and warmth as well, but if this is not possible then candles or colored lamps are good alternatives. They cast a warm light in the room, creating a very attractive ambiance and the red, yellow, and orange colors activate the lower chakras, which enhance sexual energy.

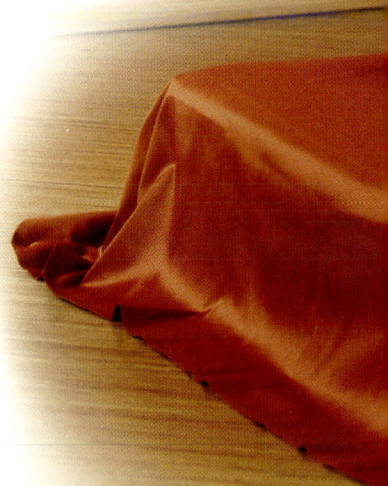

Seductive Sounds

Whether you like music as a background for erotic play and massage is something you must personally determine. Some people feel distracted by music while others love it when soft, meditative sounds accompany erotic moments.

Naturally, it would be appropriate to incorporate an element of classical Indian music—ragas, whose rich overtones often make one feel spiritual. However, Western classical music can also bring about a tranquil state of mind: works by Vivaldi, Bach, Debussy, or Ravel as well can provide a harmonic, flowing ambiance to your tantric experience, as can meditation and new age music.

Scent of Love

In order to experience the world of sensuality in all its dimensions, you should indulge the eyes (candlelight, plants, colors), ears (music), skin (silk pillows, massage oil), and especially the nose.

Essence of rose, jasmine, ylang-ylang or sandalwood are especially suited to awakening sexual energy and erotic feeling (see box on page 61). Make sure that you use only high quality oils from pure ingredients, even if they are somewhat more expensive than chemical or synthetic ones.

The application of scented oils is easy: a few drops in an aroma lamp will be sufficient. If you don't have an aroma lamp, you can put soil in a bowl filled with water and place it on a heater or use incense sticks. Remember that incense sticks vary in quality, so shop carefully. Recommended scents are rose, sandalwood, jasmine, or patchouli.

Incense is ideal for various ceremonies. In Asia, for example, it is used to drive away demons and cleanse the atmosphere. If time allows, consecrate the room you have chosen for your assignation by burning a mixture of incense and diffusing it throughout (see box on page 50).

The room in which your Tantra ritual will be held should be carefully arranged to create the perfect mood.

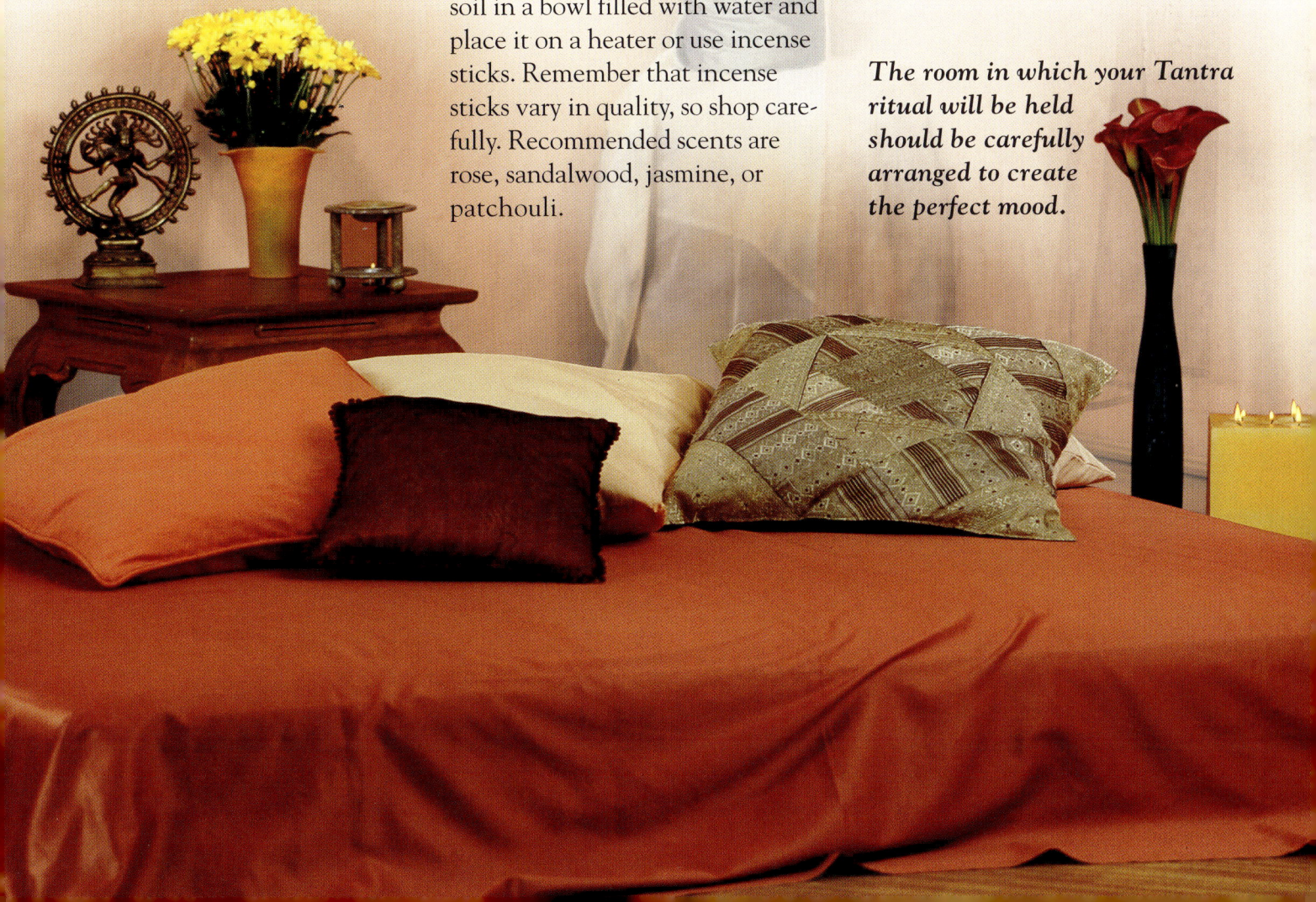

Incense For Love

Burning incense is customary in India as well as in many other cultures. Traditionally, mixtures of incense were used to drive out evil spirits, but whether these were merely representations for negative thoughts, worries, and bad vibrations

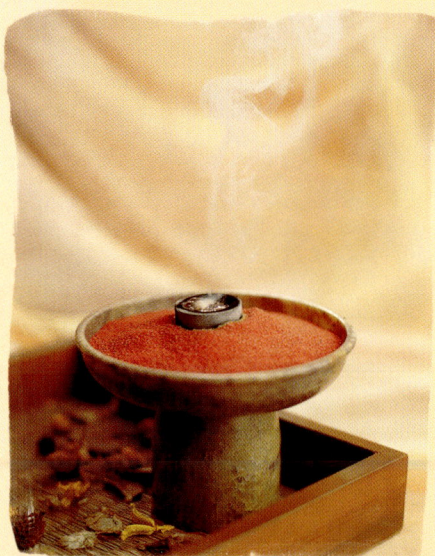

You can get accessories such as this incense burner in shops selling esoteric items.

inconducive to love is a question of interpretation.

A ritual of burning incense is simple to do and can change the atmosphere of any room in minutes. Only a few tools are required: a ceramic or metal incense dish, a fire-resistant underlay, special carbon plates to hold the incense, and a little bit of sand. These supplies can usually be found at shops that also offer packaged incense for sensuous moments.

If you would like to create your own mixture of incense, you will also need a mortar (preferably of granite or brass) to grind ingredients such as resin or bark together. Two additional tools that may be helpful are tweezers and a feather—the tweezers to hold the carbon, preventing burned fingers when you light it, and the feather to fan the aroma.

How It Is Done

First ventilate the room thoroughly to clear the air, then shut the windows tightly. Fill the incense dish with a little sand, lift the carbon with the tweezers and light it on one side, then place it in the dish. As soon as the carbon begins to crackle, gently blow on it until it is completely glowing. Put just a pinch of the incense mixture into a depression in the carbon and fan lightly with the feather, adding more incense as needed. Using your hands or the feather, fan the aroma so it envelops your partner like a bath of smoke.

Caution: To protect your furniture, place the incense dish on a fire-resistant underlay or mat and keep flammable materials such as newspaper away from the heated carbon. Always let the carbon burn out before leaving the room, or extinguish it with water. If there are children at home, they should not be allowed to play near an open flame or burning objects.

If you would like to prepare your own mixture of incense, we suggest the following recipes. (Please grind all ingredients thoroughly in a mortar).

Tantra Love Mixture I

2 parts incense
2 parts sandalwood
1 part dried rose leaves

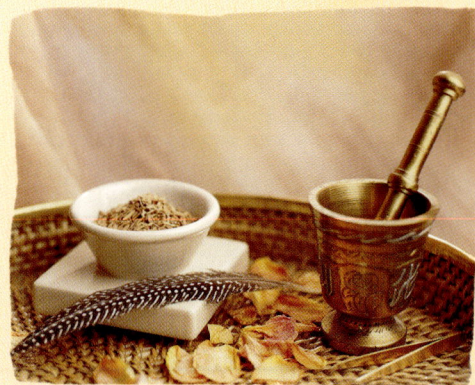

Prepare your mixture of love incense in a small mortar.

Tantra Love Mixture II

2 parts incense
1 part benzoin
1 part patchouli
1 part dried cloves
1 part dried vanilla

Cleansing and Body Care

Sensuality plays a very important role in Tantra. Therefore the cleansing and care of one's body should also become an important part of the rituals of Tantra. The tantric masters of earlier times cleansed the inner body with breathing and Tantra-Yoga techniques (see page 22) and the outer body with water and perfumed ingredients. Use heavily perfumed shower lotions and oils in moderation so your natural body smell is preserved and can enhance other scents that you may apply. Body care products with rose, rosemary, and musk are especially arousing and can be found in natural food stores.

Hygiene and cleanliness are absolute requisites in Tantra. Unpleasant smells in the mouth or body, hair stubble, and oily hair are not conducive to promoting desire and sensuality, and one can cause possible infection through unwashed hands and dirty fingernails.

You should also care for your pubic area, but do not overdo the cleansing process. Aggressive soaps affect the natural acids and oils that cover the skin and can dry the skin or create a rash. Always try to use acid-neutral soaps, especially in the pubic area.

Cleansing of Intimate Areas

During a shower or bath you can cleanse this area in a very gentle and pleasant way. Mix one cup of plain yogurt (take the yogurt out of the refrigerator at least an hour beforehand) and one teaspoon of apple cider vinegar together and apply it to your pubic area. Let the mixture work for a short time, and then rinse thoroughly with water.

Bathing Together

Those who practice Tantra find it completely natural to shower or bathe together with their partner. Wash each other's hair, then cleanse your lover from head to toe using a wash gel that is gentle to the skin. Do not neglect any part of the body, and rinse off the soap using the tingling stream of the showerhead. You can further arouse your partner by directing the streams of water onto his or her genitals or using a loofah over other sensitive parts.

After bathing, you and your partner should moisturize each other's

Mutual pleasure: bathing together.

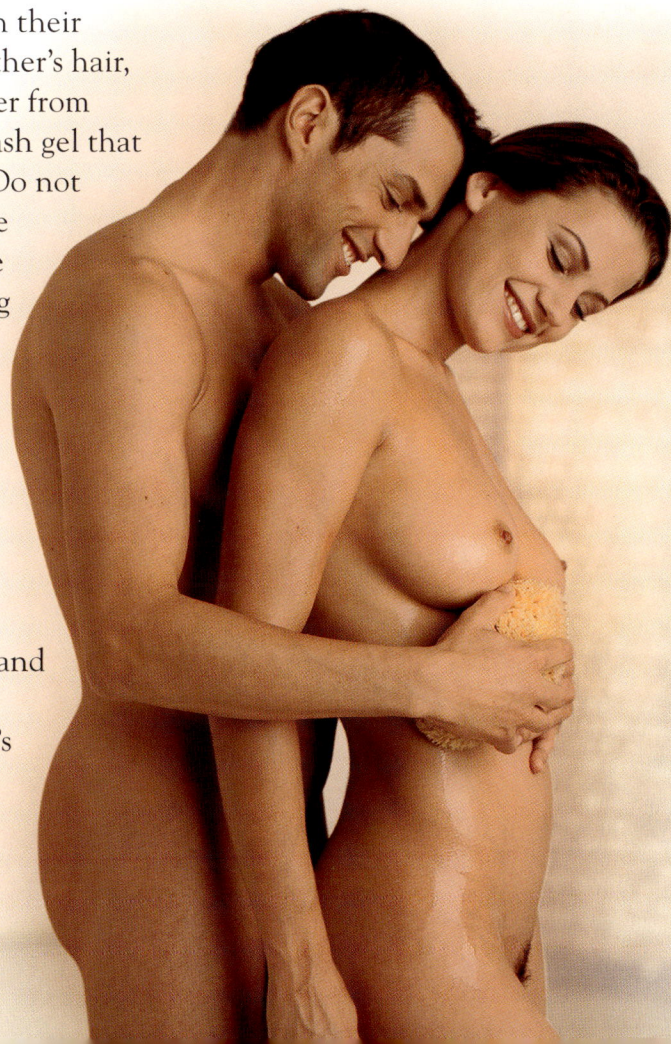

body using perfumed creams or body milk, or even perform an erotic massage (see page 60). Enter your temple of love with a thoroughly cleansed, naked body and without any distracting thoughts. Place a bathrobe or silk kimono next to your bed so if you become cold you don't have to look far for clothing.

Exchange of Energy Through Gentle Touch

The following pages introduce you to games and exercises that promote the exchange of male and female energy, personified by the Indian deities Shakti and Shiva. These exercises help you to find more pleasure and sensuality within your body through techniques that counteract inhibition and build trust.

"Shiva and Shakti Greet One Another"

While naked, place yourselves opposite one another at a distance of about one to ten feet and fold your hands in front of your breast with fingertips pointing upward. Look each other directly in the eyes and breathe fully so as to relax. Let your

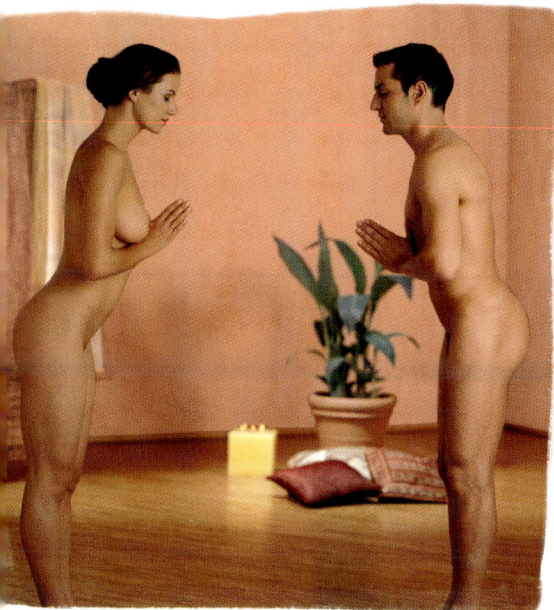

Every erotic encounter should begin with a greeting.

glance rest lovingly on the other for a time, then close your eyes and bow toward each other. This salutation shows respect to your Shiva or Shakti and exhibits a willingness to concentrate exclusively on him or her.

While bowing, imagine that you are paying homage to the male or female source of the energy you wish to connect with, who is hidden behind the external appearance of your partner.

Return to an upright position and open your eyes. Taking each other by the hand, proceed to the bedroom or area of love and continue with one of the following exercises or sexual intercourse.

The "Shiva-Shakti Game"— Giving and Receiving

The purpose of the "Shiva and Shakti Game" is to provide mutual pampering of each other—Shakti receiving what Shiva gives to her and vice versa. The game is not about reaching limits, but doing exactly what you know your Shiva or Shakti loves, then observing the reactions by following the waves of desire, facial expressions, and breathing of your partner. If you are unsure about what your partner finds most enjoyable, be sure to ask.

The easiest description of the game is that the male is the giver and the woman the receiver with, of course, the roles exchanged as the game continues. Begin with your Shakti lying in the grass or on the bed with

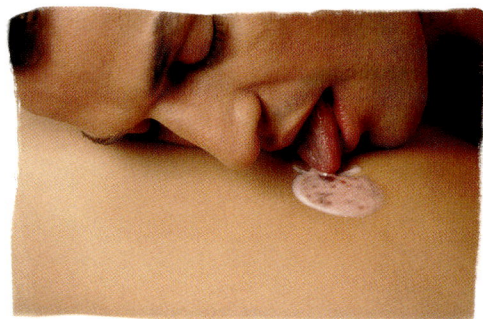

Spoil your partner with sensual games.

eyes closed and ask her to be completely passive for the next ten or fifteen minutes in order to concentrate completely on her own sensations.

While performing the exercise, both of you should remain silent, but be sure to share your experiences afterward, telling each other what you especially liked or disliked.

Decisions such as lying on her back or stomach should be made by your partner. If she is still dressed, you should slowly and gently undress her. Do not hurry, and be sure to stroke her body thoroughly after removing each item of clothing. Most importantly, be tender when exploring the body of your Shakti, imagining what you would like to do in particular.

For example, you can …

🌀 Stroke your partner's back lightly with a peacock feather

🌀 Kiss the throat of your Shakti and nibble on her earlobe or stroke her hair

🌀 Gently apply honey to her lips with your fingertips

🌀 Put strawberry yogurt in her navel and gently lick it out (if, of course, you like strawberry yogurt)

🌀 Caress her erogenous zones—for example her breasts, stomach, and the inside of her thighs (see box on page 63)

🌀 Finally bring your attention to the pubic area of your partner, called "yoni" in Tantra, and spoil her by gently kissing and stroking this area.

It is important that you thoroughly kiss, caress, and spoil your partner, but not to have intercourse with him or her. This game is about your partner's excitement, not your own.

Spoiling One Another

If the man is in the passive role, his partner should stroke and caress him, paying special attention to his "lingam," or penis. Many couples end this game by the active partner bringing the passive partner to orgasm using hands or mouth. There is nothing wrong with this as long as there is no emphasis on performance or pursuit of orgasm. Tantra views ejaculation as a waste of male energy, therefore both partners should decide at what point the game of arousal should end.

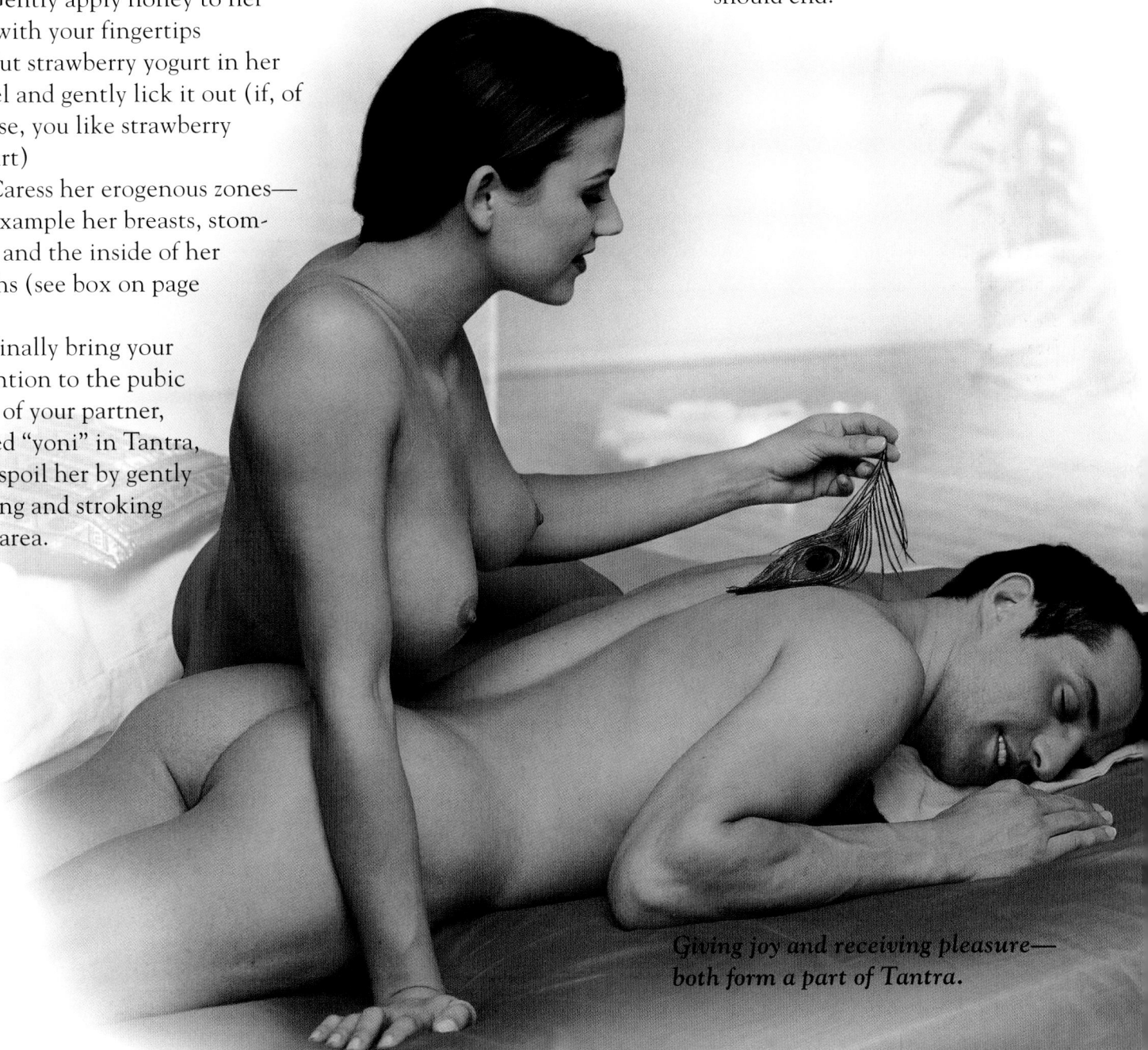

Giving joy and receiving pleasure—both form a part of Tantra.

Veneration of the Yoni and Lingam

When you give sexual satisfaction to your male or female partner, the act should never be done mechanically, but always in a sensitive and attentive manner. The penis and vagina are more than mere sexual organs: they are the center of spiritual energy and have the ability to give new life. This is the reason they have been worshiped throughout time and in many ancient cultures as the embodiment of potency and fertility. Tantra in particular has always held rituals for the worship of the yoni and lingam.

Ritual of Worship

"Lingam" is the symbol of the god Shiva. The phallus, or erect

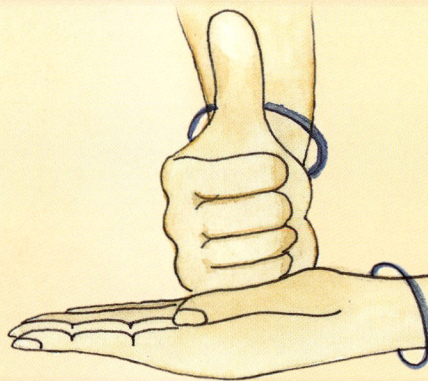

This mystical hand gesture for the lingam was used in the Odissi Temple dance.

penis, represents infinite creation and the potential for life that is found in the primal energy source of the male. In India, the representation of the

lingam was also used in conjunction with the sun and considered a powerful source of life. Worshipers carved stone phalluses for use in cult ceremonies.

"Yoni" is the term for the female genitals. The word encompasses the physical form and function of the vulva but more importantly, refers to the sacred representation of the everlasting female principle and procreative energy. The yoni is considered the womb of all creatures, the shimmering jewel as the source of all life.

In Tantra, both the yoni and the lingam were regarded as the seat of all magical power. Tantric ceremonies worshiping male and female genitalia as the source of all life demonstrated this through anointment, prostration, offerings of flowers, as well as caressing with hands and mouth. In order to pay homage to the goddess of fertility, followers of Tantra performed the "sacred yoni ritual." They poured small bowls of yogurt, honey, milk, and water over the genitals of a chosen female, then collected the liquids into a large bowl and offered it to the goddess. Each fluid sym-

Yoni and lingam united.

bolized an element of life—yogurt represented earth, honey represented fire, milk denoted desire, and oil and water symbolized heaven. The fluids, blessed through contact with

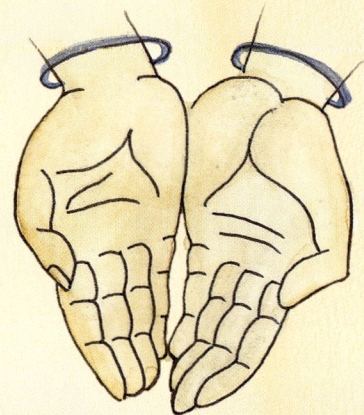

In tantric rituals, the yoni is also represented by hand gestures.

the yoni, were mixed and then drunk by the participants of the ritual. Similar rituals are also known in the veneration of the lingam.

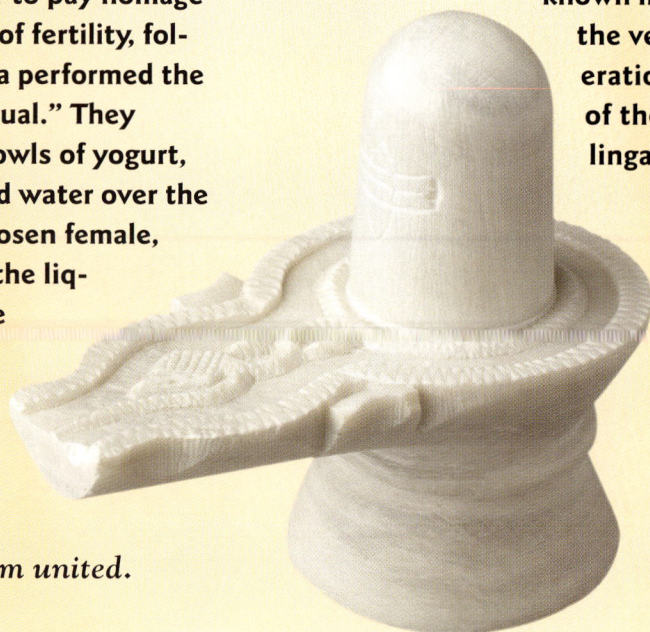

The View Into the Soul

The following exercises can help you learn to see your partner in a different and intense way. While new lovers still have the novelty of a new relationship to stimulate their passion, those who have lived together for some time often have the tendency to regard each other perfunctorily. In order to recognize the godlike potential within your partner, you must again learn to look comfortably deep into each other's eyes.

Sit down in your beautifully decorated temple of love and adjust the lighting so it is restful. Sit opposite one another, preferably in a cross-legged or lotus position (see page 30), knees just touching. Hold each other's hands, letting them rest comfortably within the grip of the other.

Finding Your Center Point Now look directly into one another's eyes, making every effort to avoid facial expressions. Take a deep breath, concentrate on your center, and look at your partner with awareness. In our society, direct contact is widely avoided because it is interpreted as a sign of physical aggression—a person in a superior position looking directly at a subordinate who in turn averts his gaze to avoid provocation.

However, Tantra propounds the idea of lovers meeting each other equally. Confidence in one another as well as mutual respect make it possible for both to gaze securely into the eyes of the other for long periods of time. Perform this exercise long enough so that you are able to see the depth and tranquility concealed within your partner.

Try this repeatedly between pauses of relaxed breathing, and give yourself over to the moment.

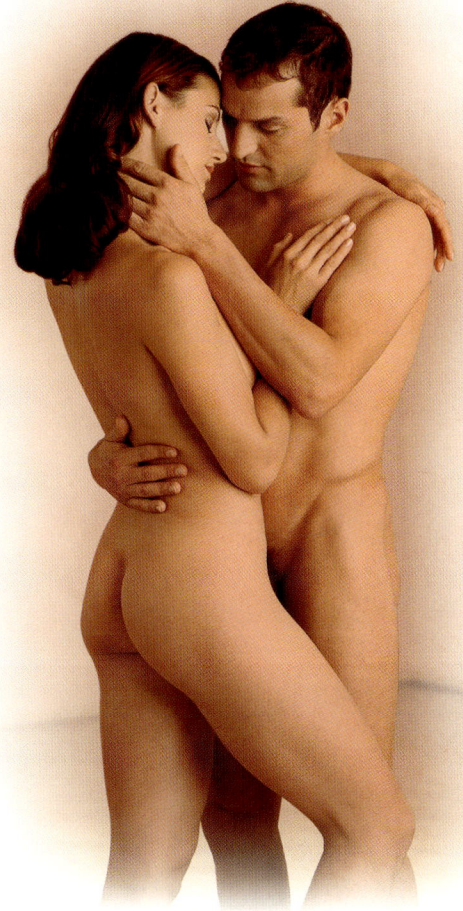

The Embrace

Embracing each other helps both partners develop trust in the other. In contrast to a quick hug, a deep embrace allows you to feel each other intensely and to feel the energy flow into each other's hearts. As an embrace continues, an energy exchange begins whereby all the chakras start to charge each other.

When you take someone in your arms you are signaling affection by offering confidence,

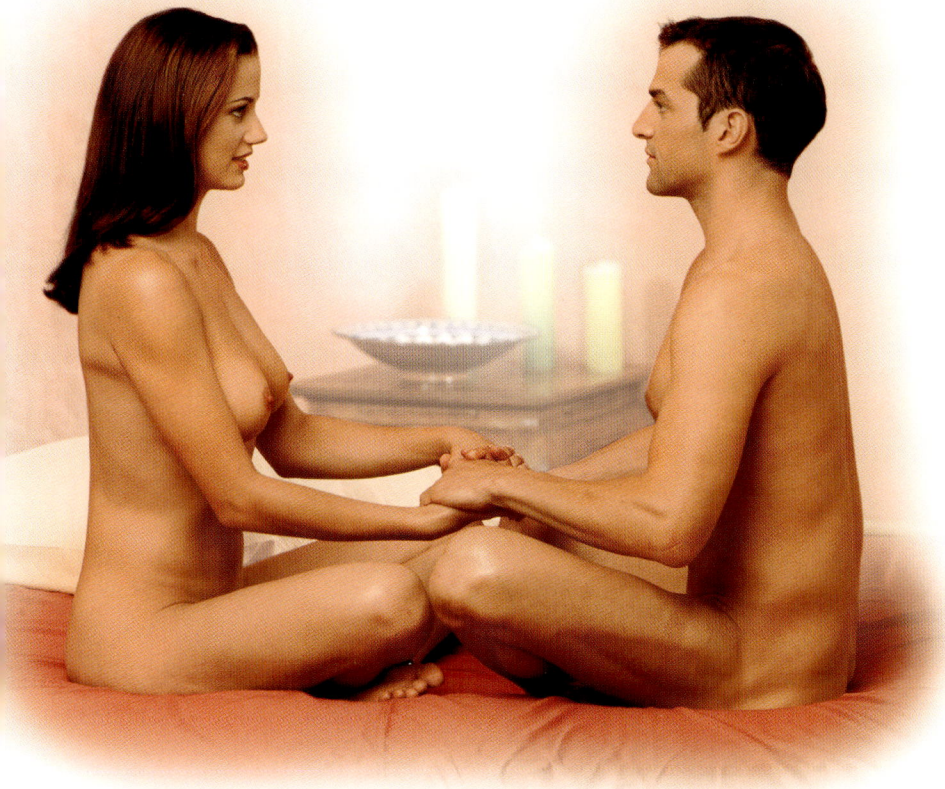

warmth, and security. An embrace has positive effects on your health, which is why you should use this form of touching as often as possible in your daily life.

To perform this exercise, it is preferable if you are both naked. Embrace your Shiva or Shakti as you would naturally, while making sure it is very close and heartfelt. Remain in this position for some minutes and observe your postures very carefully—body language often says more than verbal communication. How do you feel? Does your embrace conform to the other's body or do you establish a safe distance between each other? Do you feel gentleness and security within your partner's arms? Can

you still breathe comfortably while so close together? Be sure to change your perspective: " I embrace my lover" to "I am being embraced by my lover." Is there any time you or your partner feel reserved?

Now relax your body and breathe easily. Nestle into your partner and let the embrace begin to gently sway while you continue to hold each other. Prior to this exercise, you should decide whether to verbalize your feelings or silently follow the exchange of energy between your hearts and bodies.

"To Open the Heart"

"To open the heart" is a vigorous technique in which prana—cosmic life energy—will be trans-

ferred. It creates a healing exchange of energy in which blocks in the channels of the astral bodies are cleared, harmonizing the flow of energy. It is also a kundalini exercise that enables the life force to flow upward through the chakras.

In the example below, the woman is in the active position while the man remains passive, roles that will be exchanged later.

Feeling the Heart Chakra The man lies stretched out on his back with eyes closed. His arms are placed next to his body, palms facing up, and he is breathing comfortably. The woman sits or kneels next to her partner and concentrates on her own breathing and back posture. When she is fully relaxed, she carefully places one hand on her lover's abdomen slightly above the lingam, touching his pubic

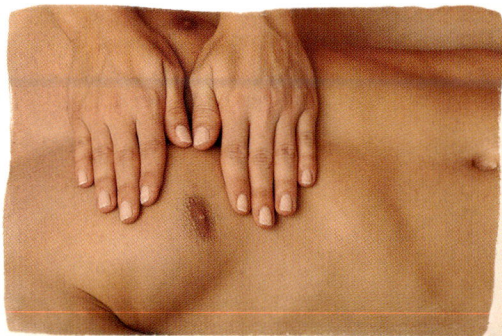

"To open the heart" at the end of the exercise, the woman's left hand slowly moves upward.

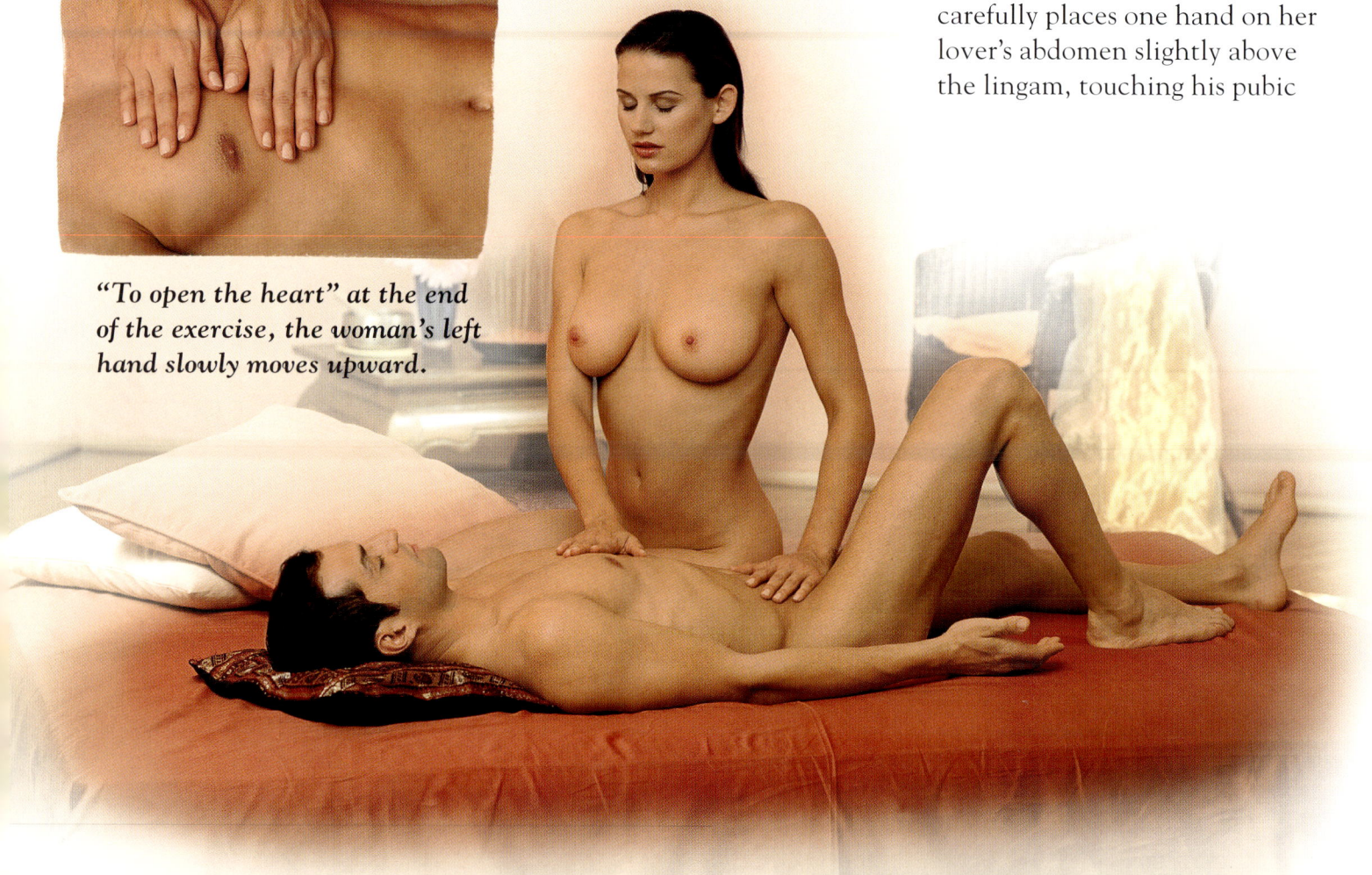

hair, and the other hand on his chest over the heart chakra.

For a few moments, the woman lets her hands passively rest on his body. As she feels the rise and fall of her partner's breathing, she also tries to feel the energy of kundalini, which rests at the base of his spine. Using the bottom of her hand, she begins to make light, vibrating motions on his body while visualizing awakening the energy in his pelvic floor.

At the same time, the man visualizes a bright, reddish beam of light flowing upward from his lower spine toward his heart chakra, where the woman's hand is resting. This ascending direction transforms the vital energy of the pelvic floor into spiritual energy that will open his heart, making it shine forth.

The exercise is finished when the woman glides her hand slowly upward along the man's torso until both hands rest in the center of his chest. Both participants should remain a short while in this position in order to feel the full effects of the exercise.

Breathing Together

The purpose of this exercise is to adjust the rhythm of your breathing so it matches that of your partner. Simultaneous intakes of breath, done slowly and calmly, increase the sense of unity and also help develop flexibility in adjusting to one another, a state that prevents conflict. Thorough relaxation

and physical and mental balance allow Shiva and Shakti to adjust their energy fields and experience identical sensations. By using synchronized breathing, many couples experience a completely new quality of shared perception.

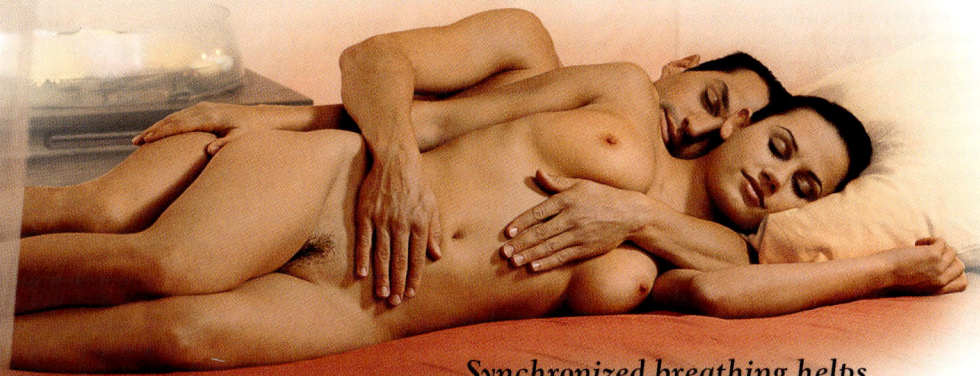

Feeling each other very closely
Lie together in the spoon position, both partners on their sides and the man behind the woman. It is important to be comfortable, so use as many pillows as needed. The man then puts his arm under his partner's head, so his hand is able to rest against her chest while his other hand is against her abdomen; in this position he is able to feel her breathing motions in both areas.

He presses his chest and abdomen tightly against her back and his legs against hers. Both partners relax as much as possible and pay attention to each other's breathing, letting it flow freely and releasing any tension with each exhalation. After some time, the man adjusts his

breathing to the rhythm of his Shakti by feeling the motions in her chest and abdomen and then inhaling and exhaling when she does.

However, this should not be done immediately. Take your time adjusting. Concentrate

Synchronized breathing helps you both experience complete harmony.

fully on your physical and mental sensations, then shut off your brain and focus on your body.

Feel your hands, chest, abdomen, legs, and how air flows in and out your nose. If you like, you may also include your hips in rhythmic breathing by gently rocking them back and forth as you breathe. Continue this exercise for at least five minutes and end it slowly. Exchange places so that the woman hugs the man from behind and repeat the exercise.

Erotic Games

The following suggestions are especially suited to relationships that may have settled into a routine and need reinvigorating.

These games inspire fantasy and provide the opportunity to try something new while testing your boundaries. Trust, love, and respect of your partner's limits are necessary conditions for all erotic games, so watch for feelings, thoughts, and resistance that may arise, and speak openly about anything that affects you or your partner. This method helps develop confidence and intimacy between you and your partner and will make it easier to avoid misunderstandings.

One thing to think about: anything that you and your partner wish is allowed in Tantra. Have no taboos or barriers in the way of your sexual ecstasy.

In these games, to trust someone else while blind is taken quite seriously.

Blindfolded

Cover your partner's eyes (with a silk cloth, for example). Unable to see, your partner becomes dependent on you; therefore, he or she must trust you and rely on your sense of touch. Use little surprises like unexpected caresses, spinning your partner around, and walking together to different places in your room. Alternate between standing very near to your partner then moving away, and watch his or her reaction.

Awakening the Senses

In order to arouse your partner's sensual curiosity, again use a blindfold and concentrate on ideas that surprise his or her sense of hearing, taste, and smell. Let your imagination run free: put drops of honey, wine, lemon juice, or yogurt on your partner's tongue, or feed your partner raisins, chocolate, or aromatic cheese. Make sounds using little bells, gongs, and drums or play unfamiliar music. You can also whisper, breathe softly, moan, or sing something romantic or daring into his or her ear, or speak very softly from across the room so you cannot be clearly understood.

Do not neglect the sense of smell: place bottles of different aromatic oils beneath your partner's nose, alternating between rose, jasmine, eucalyptus, or sandalwood incense. Other interesting possibilities are cinnamon sticks, chocolate, or anisette liqueur. Most fragrances are especially tantalizing when the eyes are covered, but be sure to pause between scents because the sense of smell can be quickly overloaded.

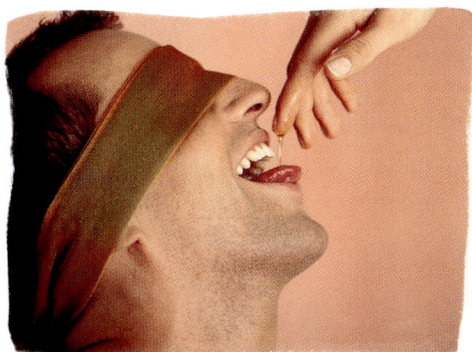

Surprise your partner with ever new delights.

The Command Game

The next game can be very informative because it brings to attention otherwise hidden preferences for sadism or masochism and dispenses with previously established roles between couples. To benefit from the game, exchanging roles is very important—each player should be both a ruler and a servant. If it has been decided that you are to be ruler first, do not forget that the tables will be turned later: and revenge can be sweet….

Develop Sensitivity Before you begin, set the rules of the game with your partner. Set it up so that for a certain time, perhaps an evening, the ruler has the power to control everything according to his or her wishes while the serving partner acquiesces without question.

To feel secure in playing this game you must have trust and affection as the underlying foundation in order to avoid unpleasantness. Developing sensitivity means getting as close as possible to the limits of your partner without trespassing those boundaries.

In playing this game, the passive partner should be blindfolded, and the ruler runs the evening according to his or her personal preferences. Be sure to exchange ideas and feelings with one another when the game has ended.

Perhaps he or she would like:

⌾ to see a naked dance or striptease performed

⌾ to enjoy a long and extensive massage

⌾ the partner in an unusual position on the bed in order to satisfy a voyeuristic desire

⌾ the partner kneeling and reciting poetry

⌾ to order the partner to masturbate—to get a few tips for future erotic games

⌾ to hear the partner sing tenderly and devotedly

⌾ the partner to leap on them in wild ecstasy

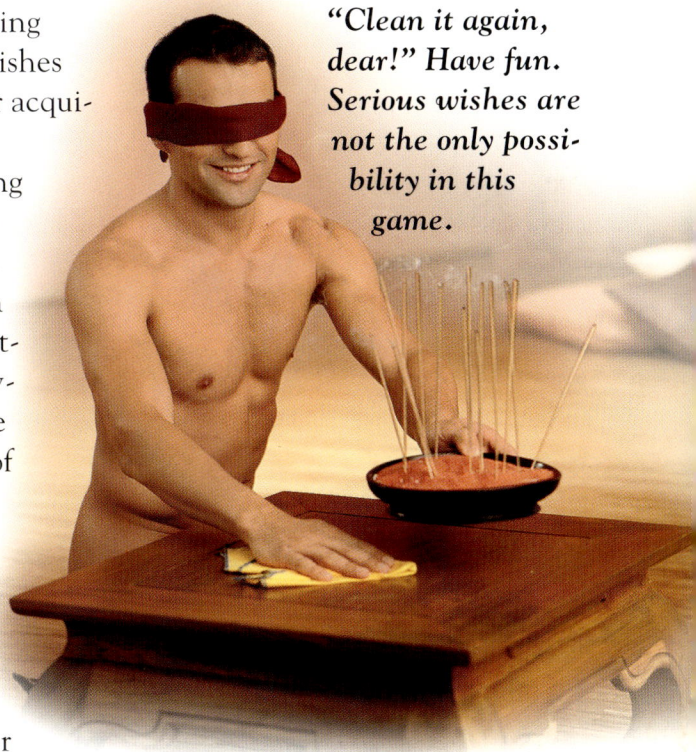

"Clean it again, dear!" Have fun. Serious wishes are not the only possibility in this game.

Having clearly defined roles in this experiment will help you think of many possibilities. The wishes you have as a ruler will tell your partner much about your secret desires. As the servant you will learn about yourself by the reactions—desire or resistance—you generate toward these wishes. You may also notice that it is easier for one partner to be in charge but more difficult to relinquish control in the reverse situation.

The most important aspect is that under no circumstances should either partner be taken advantage of; you should know each other well enough to be familiar with your partner's level of acceptance. Always respect your partner's boundaries.

Sensual Massage

Sensual massage is the ideal preparation for tantric intercourse because contact with the skin activates sexual energy and also increases desire. On the following pages you will learn massage techniques, but the most important aspect of any exercise is to pay attention to your feelings and senses when giving pleasure to your partner.

Comfortable Atmosphere It is good to use essential oils during an erotic massage because they are easy to apply and help harmonize body, spirit, and soul. The advantage of oils is that they are absorbed through both the skin and sense of smell. Inhalation of scents stimulates the brain, which in turn triggers feelings of pleasure.

Essential oils have been used for various purposes for cen-

An erotic massage is a pleasure for all the senses.

turies. In ancient India, for example, they were utilized in Ayurvedic healing processes. Today they are known to relieve pain, decontaminate and strengthen the immune system, and also lessen anxiety. Sensual benefits are relaxation and, depending on the oil used, increased desire, and fertility.

The best essential oils for sensual and erotic moments are rose (*Rosa damascena, Rosa centifolia, Rosa gallica*), pep-

per (*Piper nigrum*), sandalwood (*Santalum album*), and jasmine (*Jasminum grandiflorum, jasminum officinale*). Aphrodisiacs include ylang-ylang, cypress, and bitter orange.

The Right Mixture

Aromatic oils should never be applied undiluted because they may cause skin reactions. They are also slightly volatile and will evaporate into the air very quickly and so should always be mixed with a carrier or base oil.

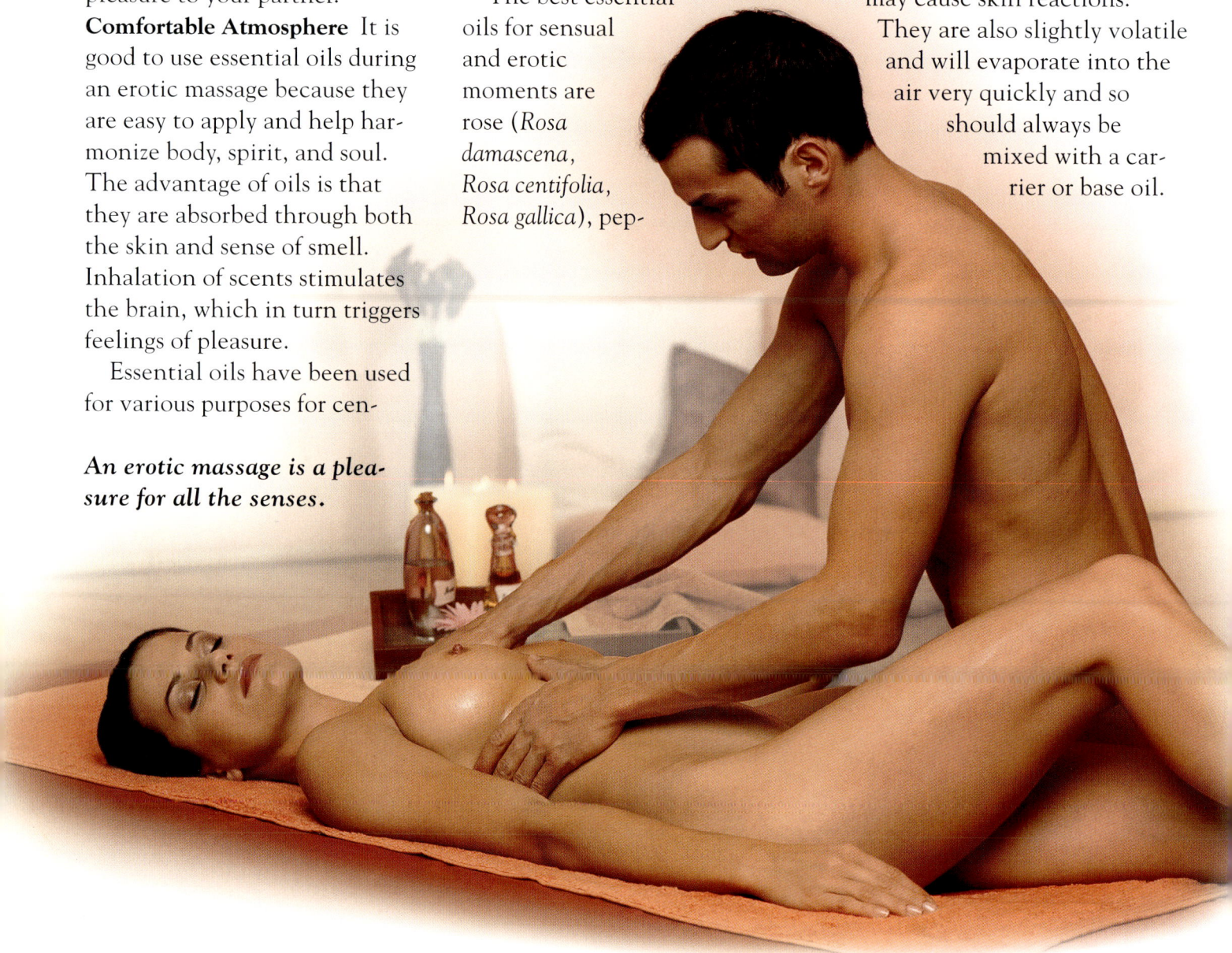

The essences can then seep through the pores of the skin into the tissues of the lymph glands, and diffuse throughout the bloodstream. Carrier oils that are especially good include avocado, jojoba, and almond.

Avocado contains many valuable vitamins and, although relatively oily, is quickly drawn into the skin. It is especially good for dry and sensitive skin.

Jojoba oil, which has been used for centuries by Native Americans, is extracted from the seeds of the desert plant Simmondsia chinesis. Chemically, it is considered a liquid wax and acts as an anti-inflammatory. It contains many vitamins and is suitable for all types of skin due to its healing properties.

Almond oil has been used as a healing and cosmetic oil since antiquity. Cold-pressed almond oil is tolerated by even the most sensitive skin and therefore is suitable for massaging the genitals. In contrast to jojoba oil, which can be stored for years, this oil should only be bought in small quantities and used immediately.

Use essential oils in small doses to avoid skin irritations; a good measure is three to four drops of essence to one tablespoon of base oil. Before using the mixture on any part of the body, test it on a small area of your lower arm for any allergic reactions. If this occurs, use a different oil.

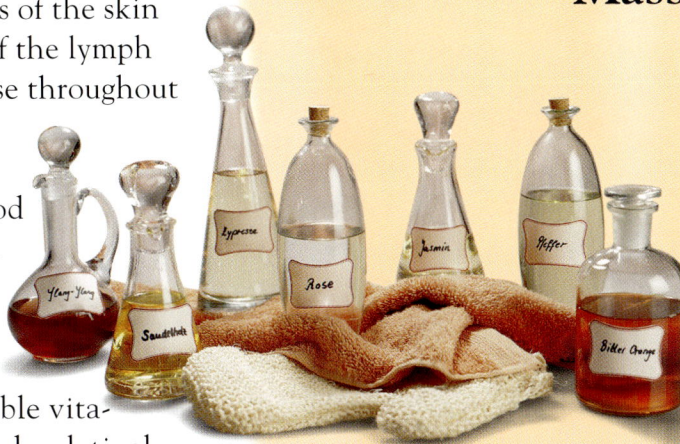

Massage Oils

You are now ready to create your erotic massage using any fragrance you prefer. The following list will introduce essences that are especially suited to sensual time together with your partner.

Rose (*Rosa damascena*) Rose oil is mainly produced in India, Morocco, and Turkey. It requires the bloom of 50 roses to extract one drop of oil. Rose is a delicate, sensual aroma that can open the chakras and release energy and rapidly create a romantic atmosphere.

Ylang-ylang (*Cananga odorata*) The blooms of this "perfume tree" exude a sweet smell immediately associated with sensuality and the erotic. This essence is especially stimulating to men.

Vanilla (*Vanilla planifolia*) Vanilla pods are grown predominantly in Madagascar. This is a classical aphrodisiac that kisses the soul and is especially stimulating to women.

Pepper (*Piper nigrum*) The oil of black pepper comes from Sri Lanka and India. It is a warm and highly arousing oil that stimulates potency.

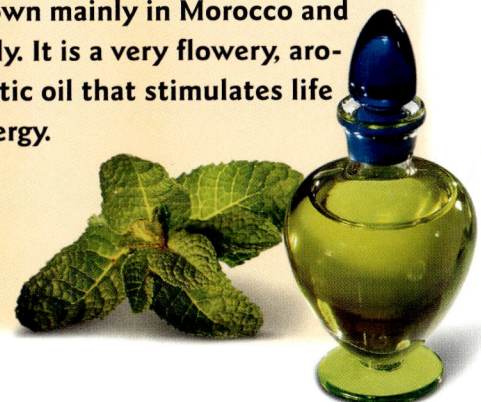

Sandalwood (*santalum album*) Sandalwood is a traditional ingredient for tantric love exercises. It creates a connection between the root chakra and crown (top of the head) chakra and stimulates the energy of spiritual love.

Jasmine (*Jasminum grandiflorum, Jasminum officinale*) In India, jasmine is known as "queen of the night" due to its hidden, almost magical way in stimulating sensuality. The oil exudes a warm, aromatic fragrance that reduces inhibition, opens the heart, and arouses desire.

Bitter orange (*Citrus aurantium*) This oil is derived from the skin of the bitter orange and has a fruity aroma that brightens your mood and brings new vitality to erotic encounters.

Neroli (*Citrus aurantium* ssp. *aur*) This oil is derived from the blooms of the bitter orange, grown mainly in Morocco and Italy. It is a very flowery, aromatic oil that stimulates life energy.

Awakening Desire With Sensual Massage

In contrast to traditional Swedish massage, sensual massage is not concerned with relaxing muscles or stimulating blood circulation. First and foremost, its goal is to awaken sexual desire through physical touch. A sensual massage should send a thrill of delight through your Shiva or Shakti and make the body more receptive to delicate contact. Therefore, you should always perform a massage very gently and with fluid movement.

Your attention should always be focused on your partner's erogenous zones. These are areas of the body that contain numerous sensory nerve endings that produce sexual excitement when stimulated by touch. They are located in different areas and are distinct from one another.

In general, women are more sensitive to touch, but the idea that men have only one erogenous zone, the

For a face massage, use only a little oil or a good face cream.

penis, is an exaggeration. It is possible to increase male and female sensitivity, and one of the best ways is with sensual massage.

Spoil Each Other In addition to the genitals, erogenous zones include the lips, ears, neck, breasts, nipples, and backside, but do not neglect the hands, feet, stomach, and inner thighs as well. These areas are all very sensitive to tender caressing. Use the following techniques, preferably in the order described. This sequence has proven successful and you can use it until you are experienced.

Face Massage

A face massage can be very relaxing since most people store a great deal of tension there The eyebrows, ears, lips, and side of the nose are part of an erogenous zone, so pay special attention to these areas. Perform this massage with slow, stroking movements of the tip of your thumb, index finger, and middle finger. Gently stroke the eyebrows and make circular movements over the temples.

Do not use essential oils on the face; use pure almond, jojoba, or avocado oils.

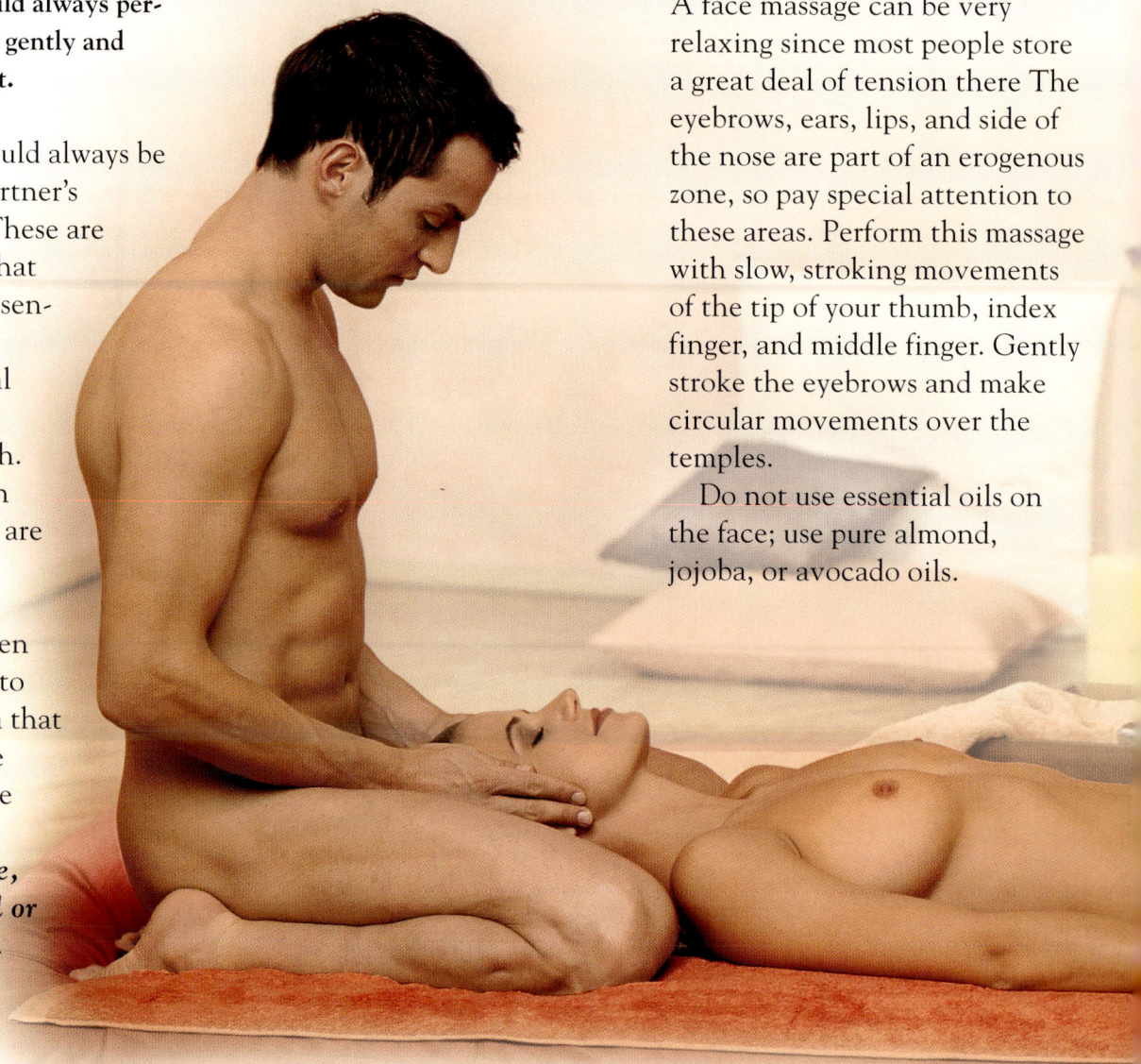

The Feet

The feet, especially the soles, are very sensitive to touch. If your partner is ticklish, avoid this area because massage would be impossible. If he or she is not, then rub the oil mixture over the entire foot. Hold the foot in your hand and stroke along the bottom, applying mild pressure with your thumb. Massage each toe individually by pulling on it gently and sliding your thumb and index finger in the space between them.

A foot massage has a very intense effect because of the many reflex zones being stimulated.

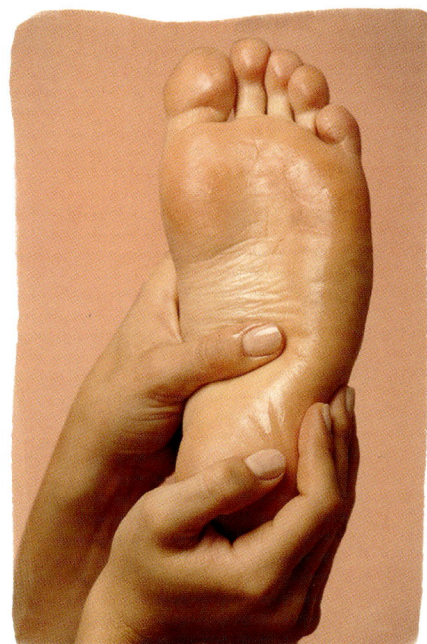

Massage Tips for Practice

It is important to have the correct ratio when mixing the base and essential oils (see page 61), before beginning your massage. But first, here are a few suggestions to make the experience pleasurable for everyone.

🔊 Perform the massage on your bed or in another open area, using a towel or sheet to rest on. Keep another small towel nearby to remove any excess oil and have a blanket ready to cover your partner with if he or she becomes chilly.

🔊 The room or area should be warm and free of drafts. Make sure your partner does not become cold since this will prevent him or her from completely relaxing. Pleasant background music can also help make the massage more effective.

🔊 Perform the massage like a ritual. Take your time. Be sure to watch your posture since the massage should be comfortable for both you and your partner.

🔊 Do not speak to each other during the massage. Concentrate exclusively on touch, breath, and the sensations created by the massage.

🔊 Warm your hands before you touch your partner's skin. Drip the oil into the palms of your hand, rub your hands together, and then spread it over the desired areas of his or her body.

🔊 Avoid essential oils when performing a face massage. Use pure almond or jojoba oil instead.

🔊 Do not massage skin that has any disease or shows varicose veins. Do not perform massage on anyone with phlebitis, fever, or serious heart disease.

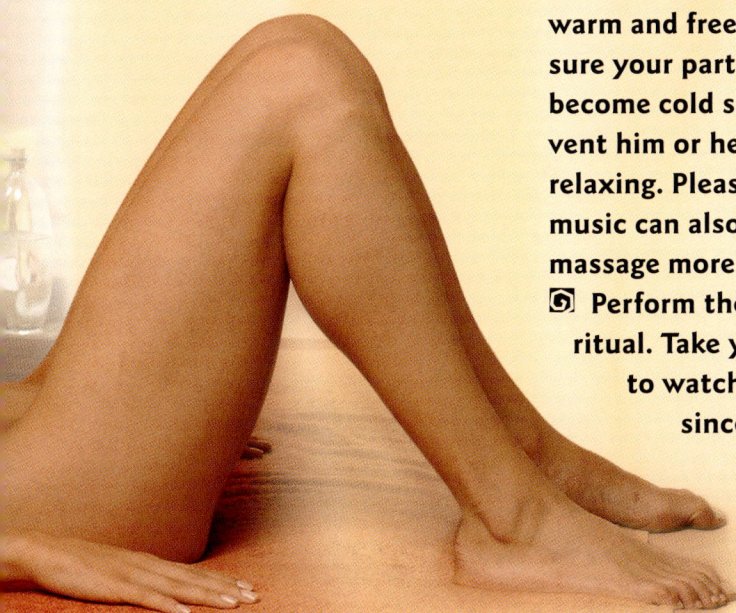

Back and Behind

The back and behind are traditional areas for massage. Here you can massage your partner a bit more aggressively to relax tension. To begin, spread the oil with regular, gliding movements known as "effleurage" over the back and behind. With your hands flat, slowly rub from the neck down the length of the back to the buttocks, intermittently using both knuckles and fingertips.

Areas that are especially sensitive are between the buttocks and the region between the backside and the upper thighs.

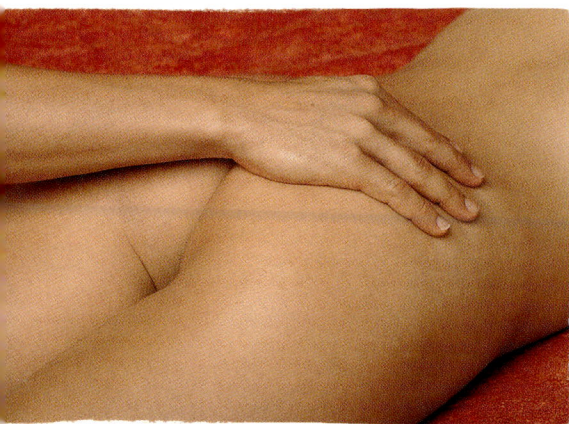

Massage the back with force, and then lessen the pressure over the lower back and buttocks.

Chest

Men as well as women respond with pleasure if the chest is gently caressed. While men can usually be massaged in this area with a bit more pressure, women's breasts should be treated very carefully.

Use a lot of oil in this area so that your hands will glide softly and easily over the skin. Make circular movements with your

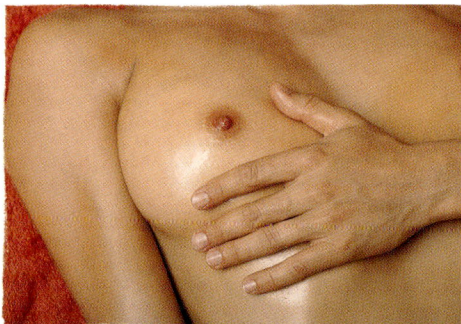

In erotic massage, caress the breasts of your female partner very softly and tenderly.

palms or draw lines over the skin with your fingertips. Do not forget to stimulate the nipples; the best way is to gently circle over and around them with the tip of your index finger.

Stomach, Hips and Thighs

After you have massaged your partner's chest, you can begin to move slowly toward the genital area. Imagine that the stomach, hips, and thighs form a ring around the genitals that you must conquer before you may advance to the center of desire.

First spread the oil around the navel. Place your hands flat on the skin above and below the navel and massage the stomach with slow, clockwise motions. Do not use a lot of pressure; rather, let your hands stroke the skin as lightly as a cat's paw.

Now move down and begin to massage the hips and thighs. Pay

special attention to the insides of the thighs, stroking upward from the knee toward the genitals. If necessary, ask your partner to spread his or her legs slightly so you can better massage inside and under the thighs.
Light as a feather In the chest, stomach, and thigh region, try a technique called "feathering" whereby the skin is only lightly brushed. With your hands totally relaxed, glide your fingertips over the skin as lightly as a

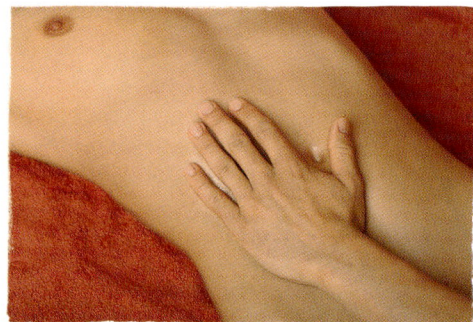

Carefully circle around the navel before moving forward to more intimate areas.

feather, alternating left and right hand.

The Yoni and Lingam

The high point of the sensual massage is the stimulation of the genitals. It is important to massage this area with great care and sensitivity.

There are several points to follow when massaging the vagina —the yoni—or the penis—the lingam. First, do not use essential oils in the immediate area of the genitals. These can easily cause irritation of the skin or mucous membrane. Use only pure base oil such as almond, which is friendly to delicate skin and will not cause adverse reactions. Be generous when applying the oil; it creates pleasurable sensations and is good for the skin.

Proceed with the massage of the yoni very carefully and watch your partner's reactions.

Be Sensuous Remember that sensual massage is primarily a preparation for tantric intercourse. This means that it is a part, but not the conclusion of the love games. The erotic hand movements described below help increase your partner's sexual energy and improve sexual awareness between you.

A woman should stimulate the perineum, testicles, and shaft and glans of the penis by first making circular motions over them with her hands. Then, using a lot of oil, she should glide her hands repeatedly over the penis.

The best way for a man to pleasure his partner is to spread oil over her entire pubic area. With the tips of three fingers, he should then smooth the oil carefully over her inner and outer labia, moving back and forth, and then spread oil over the clitoris. Being very careful, he should make circular motions, vibrating the clitoris gently.

Take Your Time Take as much time as necessary— especially when massaging the genitals. In between hand movements, watch your partner's reactions. Just as when you masturbate your partner, previously established roles can influence the effects of sensual massage. For example, one partner may automatically assume an active role while the other remains passive. Try to avoid this by taking turns in giving and receiving.

Spoil Each Other In Tantra it is important that you fully explore not only your body, but that of your partner as well. This is accomplished by giving and receiving pleasure equally.

Generally, the person performing the massage feels as if he or she is giving while the passive partner gets something, but Tantra avoids such terms because the goal is the mutual exchange of energies. If you remain relaxed and fully engaged while performing massage, you will also feel that you are getting something back.

If you receive a massage, be aware that you are giving something to your partner through your reactions. This attitude makes it possible to have a wonderful experience together.

Massage the lingam very gently at first and then with more intensity.

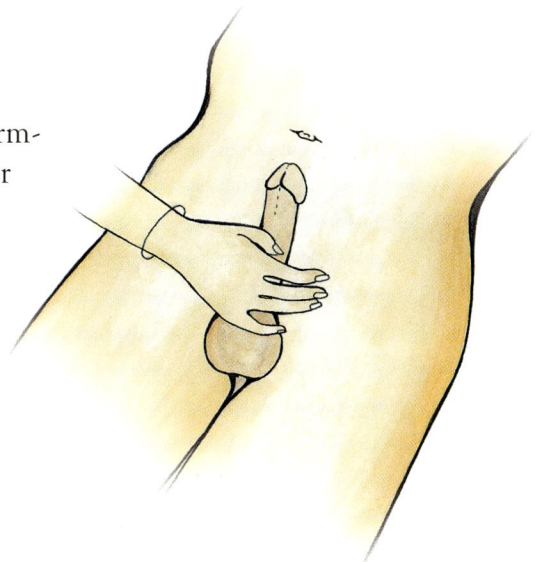

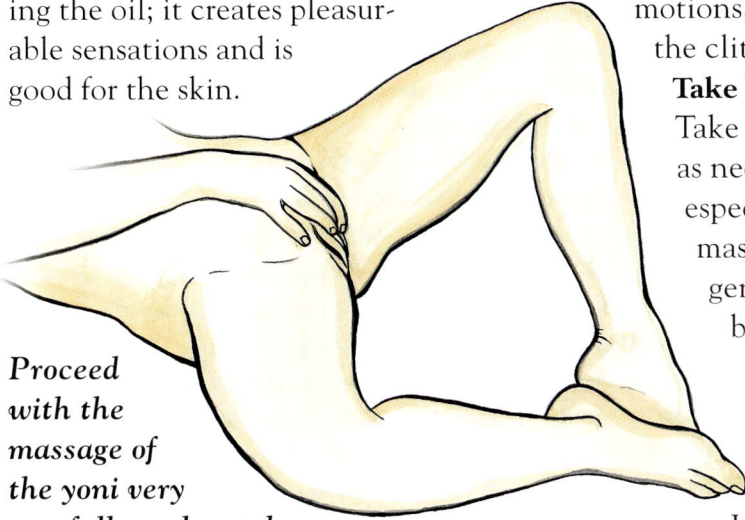

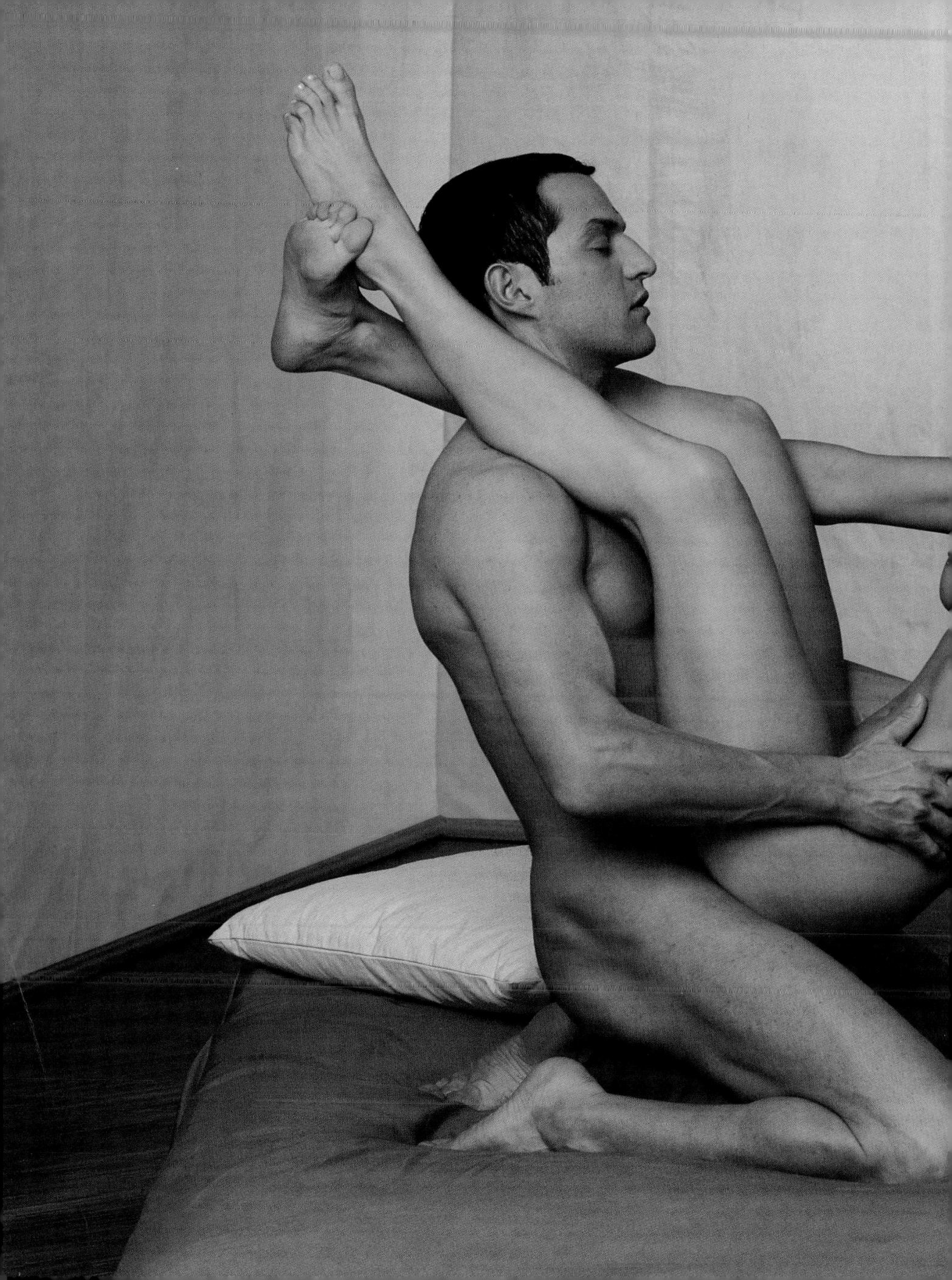

Tantric Intercourse

The goal and high point of Tantra is tantric intercourse between a man and woman; however, this type of intercourse is substantially different from the "ordinary" kind. It is not concerned with the swift satisfaction of lust, but with the expansion and sensitivity of conscious awareness. The sexual act can only culminate in a complete merging if intercourse is performed as a ritual with active engagement, meditation, and plenty of time.

Merging Together

Tantra is not only concerned with physical intercourse between a man and woman, but also the merging of spirit and soul. While the discipline does promote the use of exotic positions to enhance sexual pleasure, Tantra's ultimate purpose is the total unification of partners.

The purpose of Tantra-Yoga techniques, sensual games, and erotic massage is the preparation for tantric intercourse. Now, in the following pages, you will learn about the traditional positions used in intercourse, which derive from the main writings of Tantra, the *Kama Sutra* and *Ananga-Ranga*.

Similar to Yoga *asanas*, all the tantric positions build on one another. Because they are progressive, they should be practiced in the order given, and they should be practiced with meditative concentration. Do not begin with the most difficult position first; you may not be mentally or physically prepared for it.

When you and your partner first begin, limit yourself to one or two love positions per Tantra session. Later on you and your partner can change positions more

often, but you should always do so smoothly and slowly.

Inner Focus Besides enhancing sexual intercourse, tantric positions serve to increase flexibility of the muscles and tendons and improve oxygen supply to the cells. Tantric positions also have a beneficial effect on blood flow to the inner organs.

The spiritual aspect of Tantra is just as beneficial as the physical and perhaps even more important. While the sex act concentrates on the body and physical sensations, Tantra directs attention to the inner ethos; the merging of man and woman occurs in heart, soul, and spirit. Combined with energy exchange and activation of the chakras, heightened awareness can lead to exceptional sexual ecstasy.

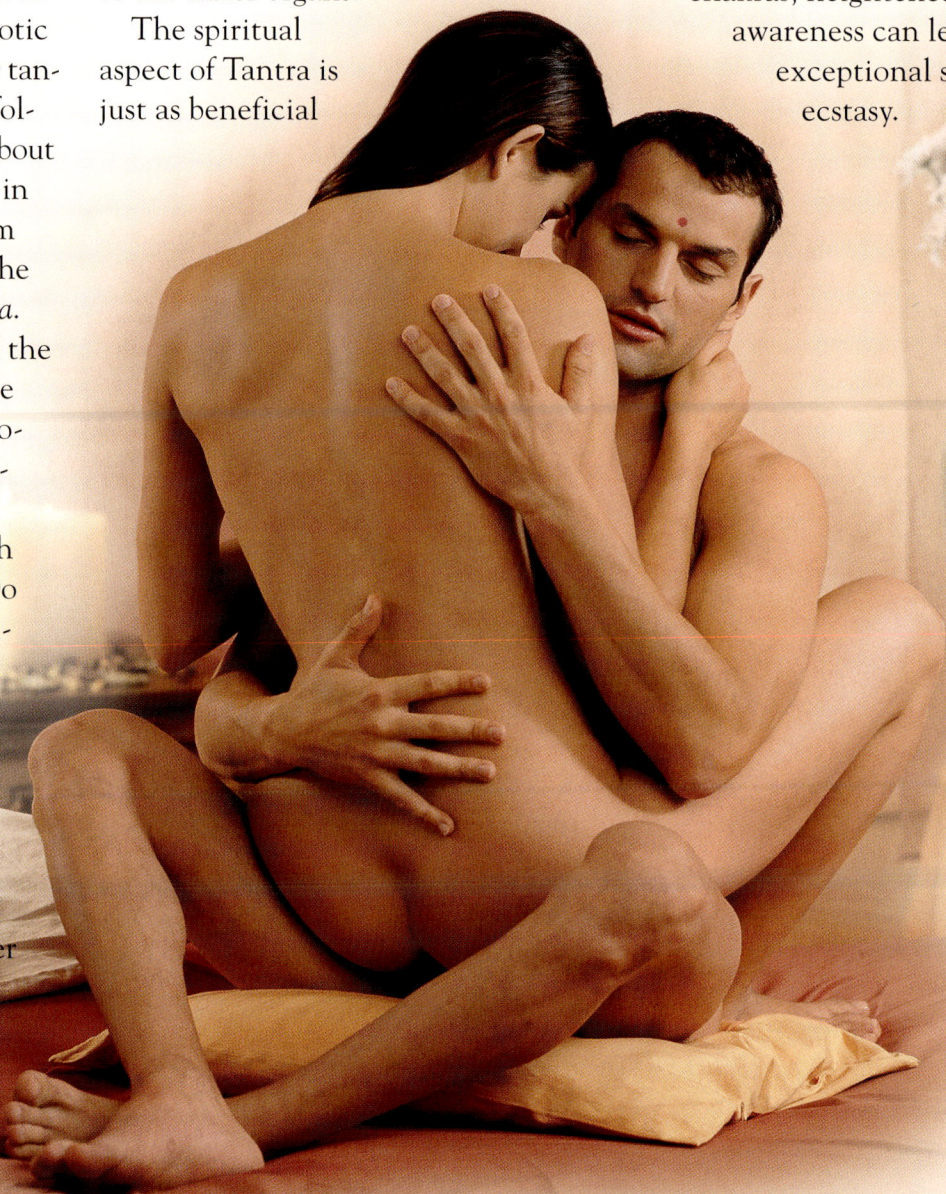

Abandon yourself to conscious intimacy.

The Tantra Ritual

There are many ways to ritualize tantric intercourse. Together with your partner, develop the one that is best for you.

Tantra rituals can be very varied. They can be performed in the presence of a guru or alone; they might involve a group, or they might be an intimate twosome; they can last several days or merely one hour; and they can have detailed rules or be absolutely free of instruction.

How you perform your tantric ritual should be decided between you and your partner but keep in mind that the philosophy of Tantra promotes the joy of life; therefore, control or rigorous rules are inappropriate. The difference between routine coitus and tantric merging is the atmosphere, conscious awareness, time and, most importantly, the intimate rites you and your partner decide upon.

Atmosphere You have already seen ways in which you can create a sensual temple of love in the chapter "How to Evoke a Tantric Atmosphere" (see page 48). Through scent, music, color, lighting, temperature, flowers, soft blankets, and pillows, you have the ability to change the sexual ambiance of any room.

Inner Consciousness It may be surmised that you already have inner consciousness, otherwise you would not have chosen this book with the goal of intensifying your sex life! You now know that Tantra-Yoga, breathing techniques, and games prepare body, soul, and spirit for Tantra, but you must also be aware of the cosmic principles that sexual desire is based on. Meditation on these principles contributes to inner consciousness and the dissolution of duality through intimate merging.

Arrangement and Timing Even though you should be creative and experiment with different ways of arranging your Tantra ritual, it might be helpful to have a few suggestions at first. There is only one rule concerning the amount of time a tantric ritual takes—the longer it takes, the better.

Your Ritual Can Look Like This

It is imperative that you allow enough time for your ritual! The minimum is an hour, but it is far better to reserve an entire evening for Tantra.

Some couples prefer love in the morning while others prefer the evening or even the middle of the night. On weekends or vacation, you should experiment with different times to find whether Tantra in daylight or in the moonlight suits you best.

Whatever you decide, remember the importance of not rushing.

Prepare some symbolic objects for your game of love:

- A holder with two burning candles
- Two beautiful glasses
- A carafe with fresh water
- A small carafe with red wine
- A piece of bread

You may also want to add some fish or a piece of meat. Don't take time to cook, merely add some smoked salmon and

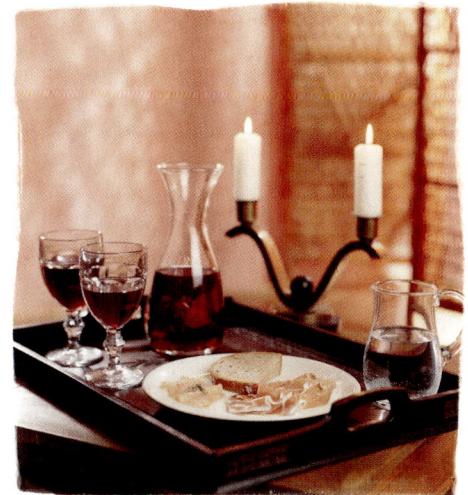

Create the proper mood for your amorous encounter.

slices of ham; the purpose is not to fill your stomach, but to provide symbolic representation. For example, wine symbolizes the fire of passion, meat symbolizes air, fish is naturally water, and bread is the earth. The two burning candles are symbolic of the light of both souls who have found each other and unite together through tantric intercourse.

Spoil Yourself If you have eaten, be sure to wait at least two hours until you begin your ritual. Then begin by bathing together with your partner, slowly soaping each other generously, and then drying and moisturizing each other with a fragrant cream. Proceed with a sensual massage (see page 60).

Look Into the Soul While still naked, take each other by the hand and silently enter your room of love. Stand opposite each other, bow deeply, and perform the greeting (see page 52). Now sit on the floor in a comfortable Yoga position and, while clasping hands, stare deeply into each other's eyes for about a minute (see page 55). At an agreed signal, both should chant the mantra *om* three times—first for the cosmic goddess, the everlasting female principle; second for the cosmic god, the everlasting male principle; and last for the universal unity that can be attained through intercourse.

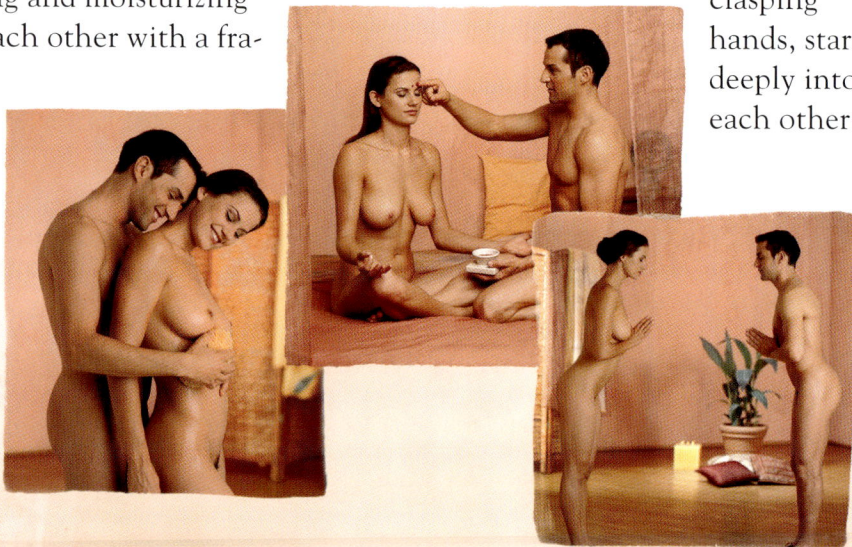

The Third Eye Now the man will softly chant the mantra *om nahma Shaktia* as he draws a red dot in the middle of the forehead of his Shakti in order to mark the third eye, or point of cosmic awareness (henna or kum-kum powder is best for this purpose).

In this manner, the man greets his beloved and consecrates her for intercourse. When he is finished, the woman then chants *om nahma Shivaya* three times as she proceeds to draw a similar dot on his forehead (for mantras, see box at right). In unison, they perform the breathing technique "Awakening Kundalini" (see page 34), then drink some water and wine and partake of the fish, meat, and bread.

Now lie together on your bed or in your meadow and begin to kiss and caress one another, sleep with one another, and enjoy the peak of the *maithuna* ritual.

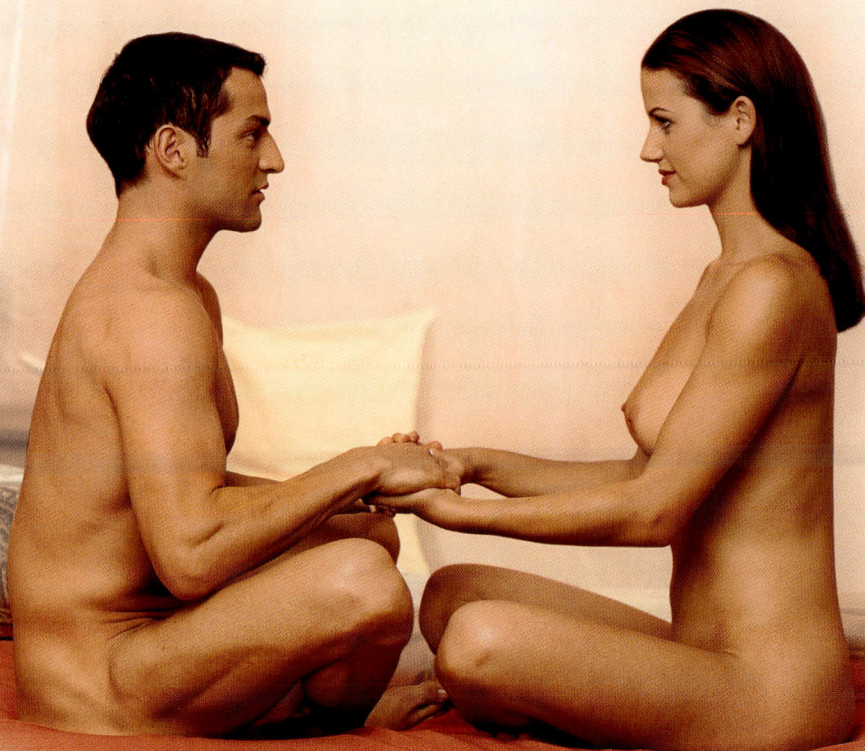

Create the proper mood for your amorous encounter.

Sexual Positions

You and your partner should determine which Tantra positions best correspond to your personal situation and should always be willing to sample something new.

On the following pages you will learn the most important Tantra positions. Start with the easiest and most comfortable postures and find those that give you and your partner the most pleasure. Don't forget to experiment! Positions in which the man is always on top of the woman offer little room for playful research; allow the woman the freedom to take control by sitting or lying on top of her partner.

Other possibilities include lateral positions, which are probably the most comfortable and back-friendly; sitting positions, which promote the highest level of engagement and awareness and are frequently used in Tantra; and standing positions, which are somewhat the exception but can be performed by a strong male with a light partner.

Often the roles in a partnership become stuck in the familiar. For example, a man might feel that he can only find pleasure if his partner lies on her stomach. If you find an emphasis on a limited number of positions, it is very important to break

these patterns and explore new possibilities. Always talk to your partner about feelings or moods that specific positions create.

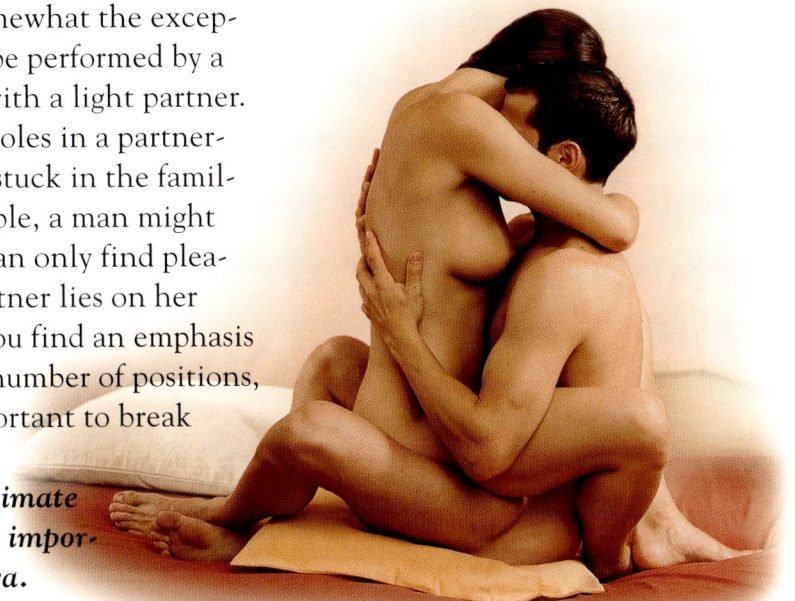

Close and intimate fusion is very important in Tantra.

Mantras

Mantras are mythic formulas; they are invocations or incantations. Most have no direct meaning but are powerful due to their energy-expanding vibrations. Mantras are used in meditation. Tantra uses mantras to evoke a specific atmosphere, which calls forth special physical and spiritual reactions.

Om is undoubtedly the best known of all the mantras. It is a universal chant that produces tranquility and concentration, but it is also used in other forms. The man, for example, greets his

female partner with the greeting *om nahma Shaktia* while the woman uses the form *om nahma Shivaya* to greet her male partner. It is enough to say all the mantras very softly, but you should draw out the vowels in a relaxed tone when you are chanting.

Two other mantras are important in Tantra: the first is *om adi om* and can be used when you want to arouse desire, for it is truly sexually stimulating, especially if you simultaneously focus your awareness on your genitals.

Repeat the mantra as you picture a sensual scene or envision an erotic fantasy (in Tantra, mantras have additional symbols, the so-called yantras).

The second mantra, used when you are establishing erotic contact, is *pa da oman*. In contrast to the former, this mantra is used to moderate your excitement if you are coming too quickly to orgasm. Repeat the mantra several times to yourself while concentrating on your heart chakra, located in the middle of your chest.

Uttana

Positions associated with the term *uttana* are ones in which the woman lies on her back. In addition to the well-known missionary position, other variations of this posture include the man kneeling before his lover or lying directly on her in order to penetrate her.

Wide-Scissor Position

The man kneels or sits in front of his lover, who opens her legs similar to the opening of a scissors: one leg bent at the knee remains lying on the bed while the other rests on the shoulder of her partner. The man moves the

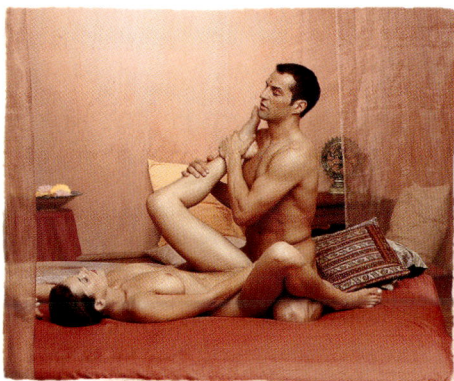

The male is the active partner in the Wide-Scissor position.

legs slightly more apart while gently squeezing the ankle of the leg resting on his shoulder.

Tight-Scissor Position

The man kneels or sits in front of his partner, whose legs are placed in a modified Wide-Scissor position with her legs closer together. The leg on the bed remains straight and touches the waist of the man. He can then lovingly caress the breasts or thighs of the woman.

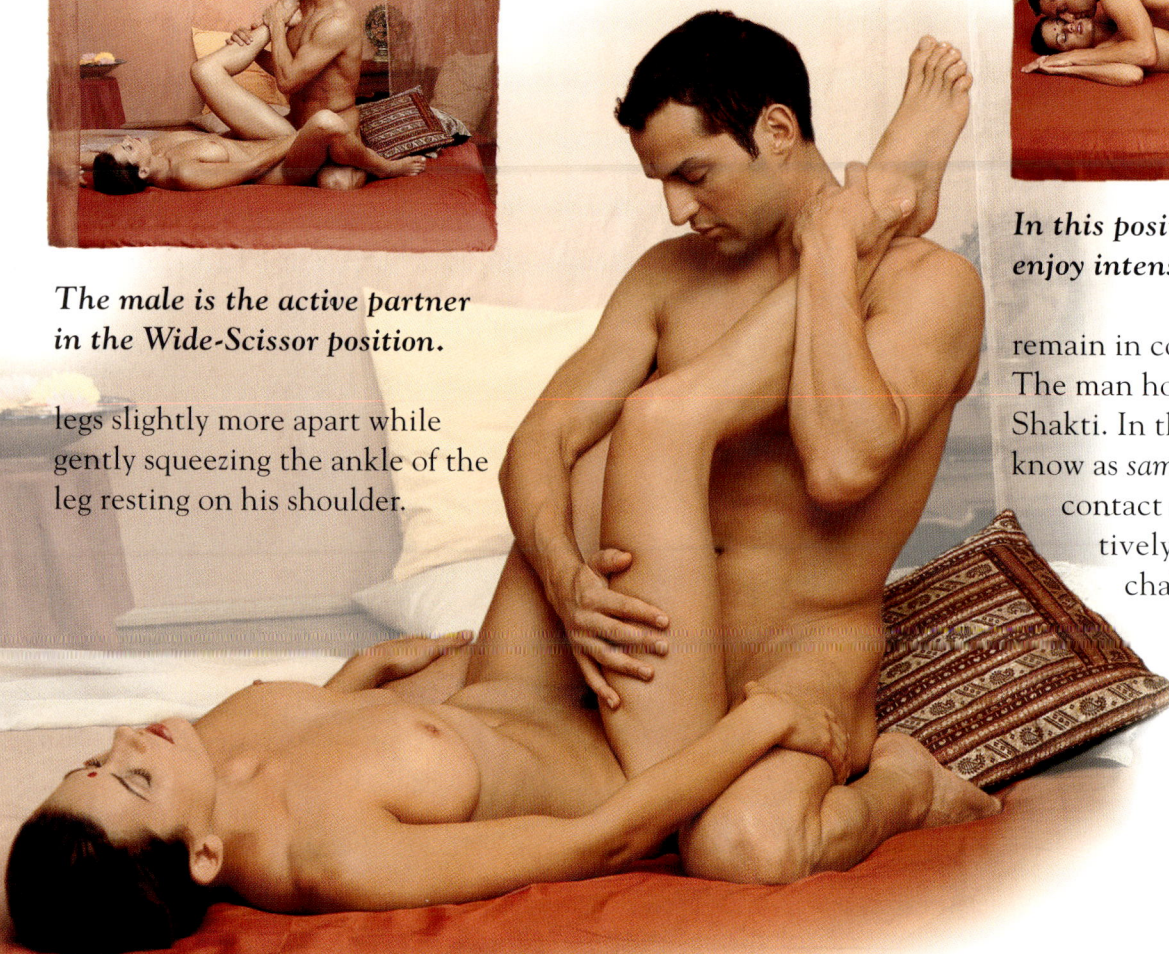

Open Rose Petal

Lying on her back, the woman opens her legs and extends her arms above her head. Her partner lies directly on top of her outstretched body, legs slightly spread so that their thighs

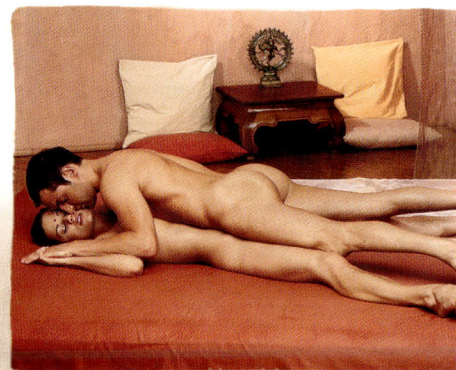

In this position both partners enjoy intense skin contact.

remain in continual contact. The man holds the hands of his Shakti. In this posture, also know as *samarachak*, the intense contact of skin will effectively activate the chakras.

In the Tight Scissor position, the woman abandons herself completely to her lover.

The Open Swing

The starting posture is similar to that of the Half Moon Position (see right), except that the woman places her feet on the shoulders of her partner rather than against his chest. Her legs are spread far apart in order to facilitate penetration. In this position, contact and friction between the penis and vagina are generally less intense.

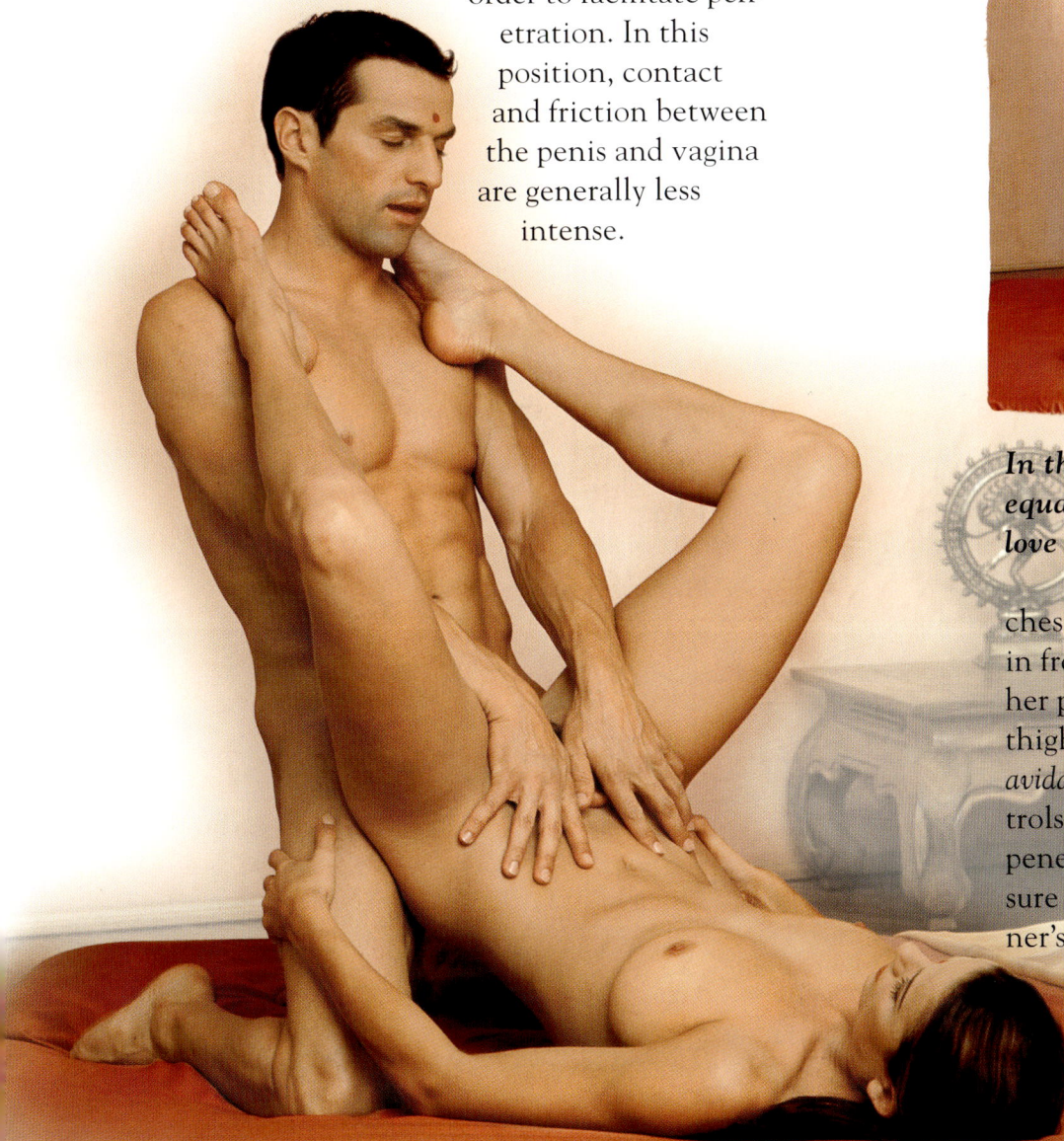

Half Moon Position

While lying on her back, the woman bends her legs, pulls her knees toward her chest, and places her feet on her partner's

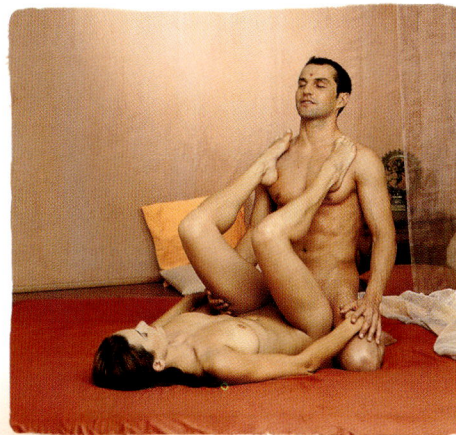

In this position, both partners equally control the intensity of love play.

chest. The man kneels directly in front of her and either holds her pelvis or grasps her ankles or thighs. In this posture, known as *avidaritha asana*, the woman controls the depth and movement of penetration by varying the pressure of her soles against her partner's chest.

In this position the man is able to gently caress his partner with both hands

Closed Swing

This position is a variation of the "Open Swing," in which the woman places her calves over the shoulders of her partner and extends her pelvis in an upward motion. Her back has to be very flexible, and to prevent any discomfort of the spine, the man should avoid leaning forward.

To make this position more comfortable, a pillow should be placed under the pelvis of the Shakti.

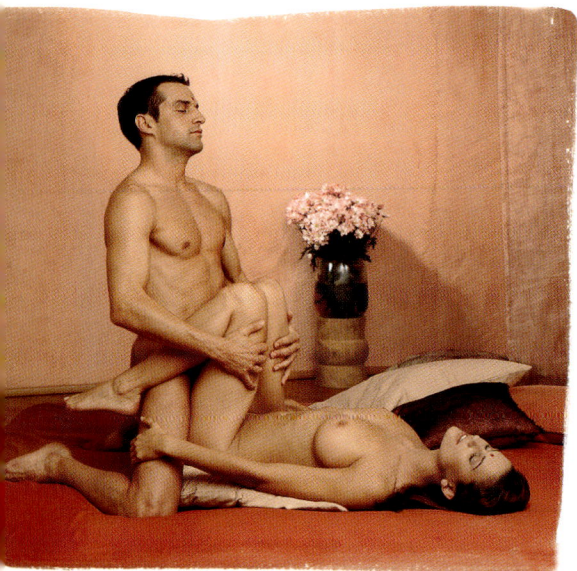

The lovers are able to feel each other with great intensity.

Sitar Position

The man kneels or crouches before his partner, who is reclining on her back. As he enters her, she closes her legs and stretches them upward. To make this position easier, Shakti can lean her legs against the upper body or shoulders of her Shiva. The Sitar Position enables deeper penetration but limits the woman's freedom of movement; the man becomes the sole active partner.

Lingam Press

In this position, the woman lies on her back with her legs drawn up to her chest. Her partner kneels between her legs and, as he penetrates her, squeezes her thighs together. This action allows both partners to experience the acute feeling of contact between the lingam and yoni. The woman can enhance the feeling by strongly and rhythmically contracting the musculature of her vagina. This position, known as *sputhma bandha*, allows men with smaller penises to feel deep penetration. The lingam press is not recommended for men who ejaculate quickly.

Missionary Position

The Missionary position is well-known to most people and is a traditional tantric posture called *saumya bandha* in Sanskrit. The woman lies comfortably on her back and, as the man reposes between her legs, she places her legs around his thighs or backside.

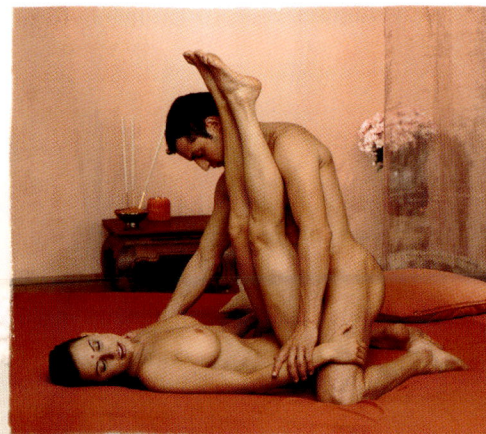

The woman abandons herself completely. Her lover can penetrate her deeply.

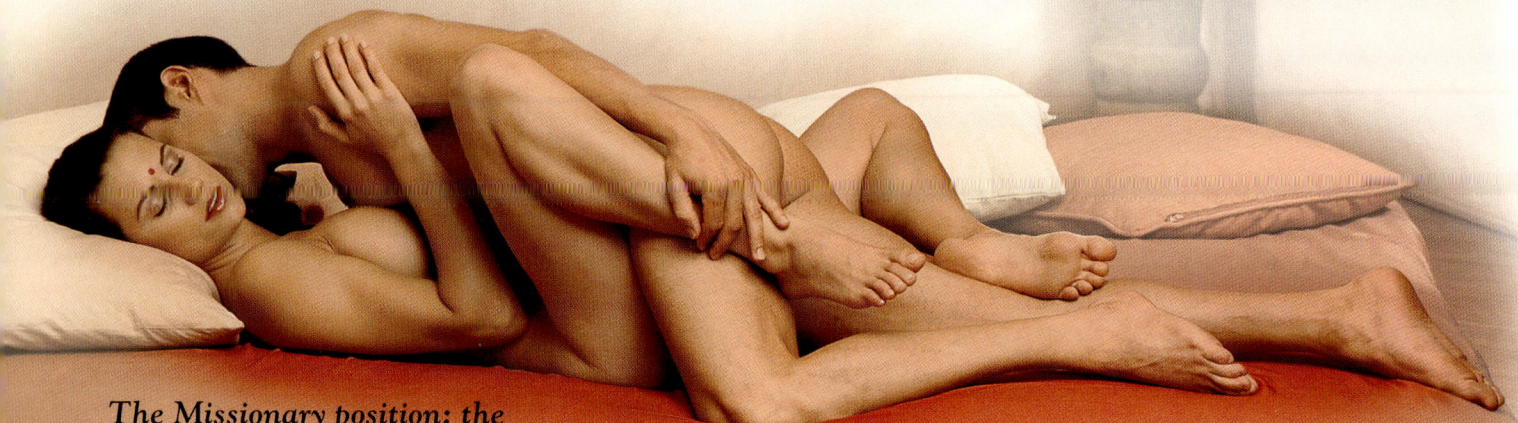

The Missionary position: the classic position of love.

Devotional Yoni

In this position, the woman proffers her yoni to her lover with devotion, meaning that she opens herself completely to him. Lying on her back, she draws her knees toward her chest and, grasping her calves or ankles with her hands, widely spreads her legs. If she is very agile, she should attempt to lay her thighs next to her pelvis. The man then kneels before her and takes control. The devotional yoni can be very pleasurable for the woman because the clitoris is vigorously stimulated.

In this position, the woman enjoys being spoiled by her partner.

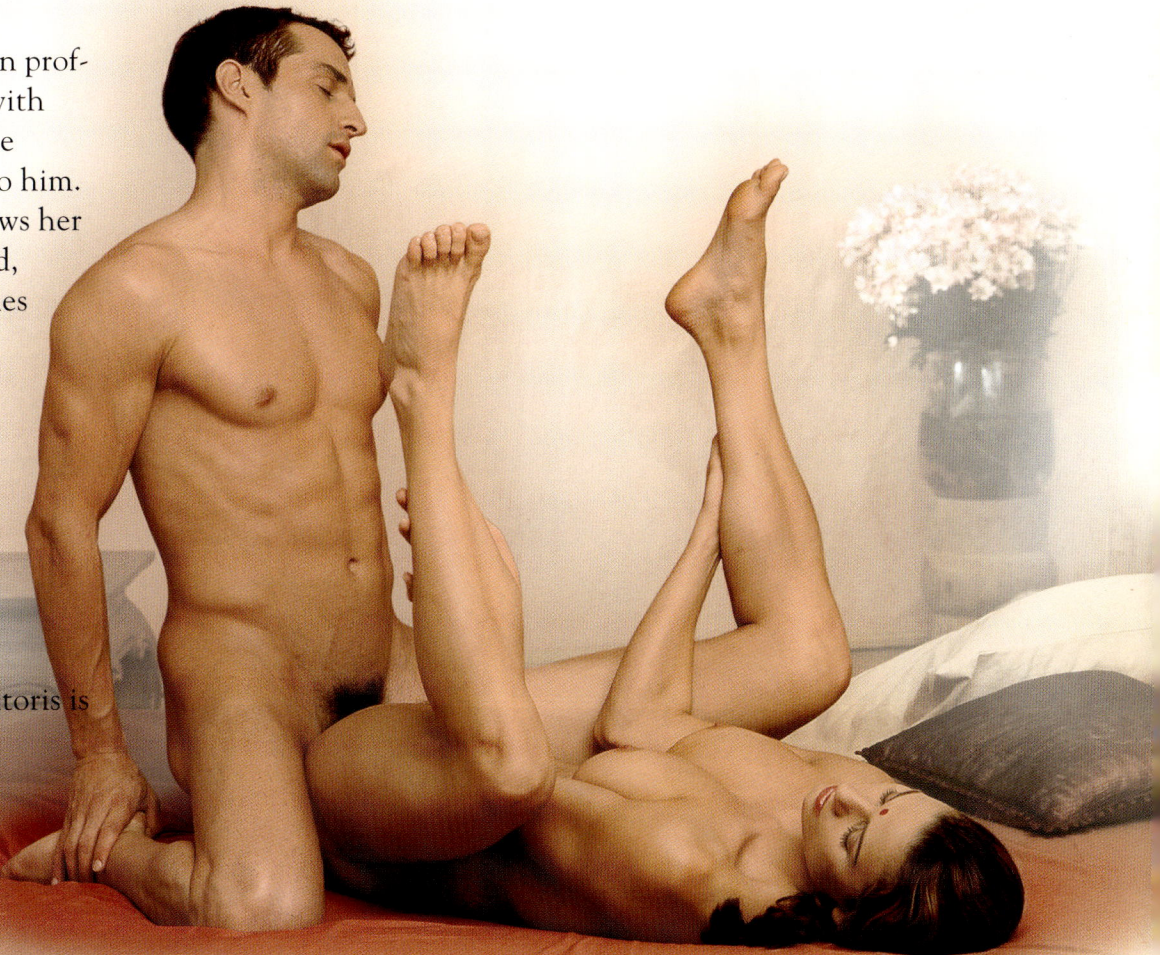

The Pressing Mare

This position, also known as *puhapakad*, is useful to partners who have either a stretched vagina or a small penis. Lying on her back, the woman opens her legs wide to make penetration by her lover possible. She then brings her legs close together in order to press her partner's penis intensely. The man lies flat on top of his Shakti with his legs outside hers. He holds his partner's hands or, to allow more movement, supports the weight of his upper body.

In this position the male feels his partner more intensely.

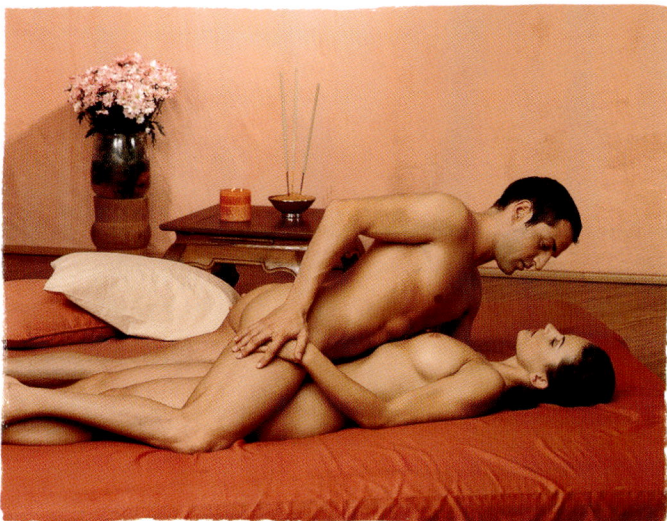

Vyata Asana

In the sexual positions described here, the woman lies before her partner on her abdomen or knees. For her, a feeling of trust and surrender will be especially strong, which may be an additional attraction in your love games.

Closed Tiger Position

The woman kneels in front of her partner with her legs together as the man kneels behind her, legs comfortably spread to maintain contact with her body. Contact between the penis and vagina is as intense as in the Open Tiger position (see below), but the man is not able to penetrate as deeply.

spine straight which is not as stressful as lying forward (see below). This also makes it easier for her partner to caress her breasts thoroughly.

Variations

In both Tiger postures, the woman can support herself on her elbows rather than placing her head and upper body on the bed. In this manner, she keeps her

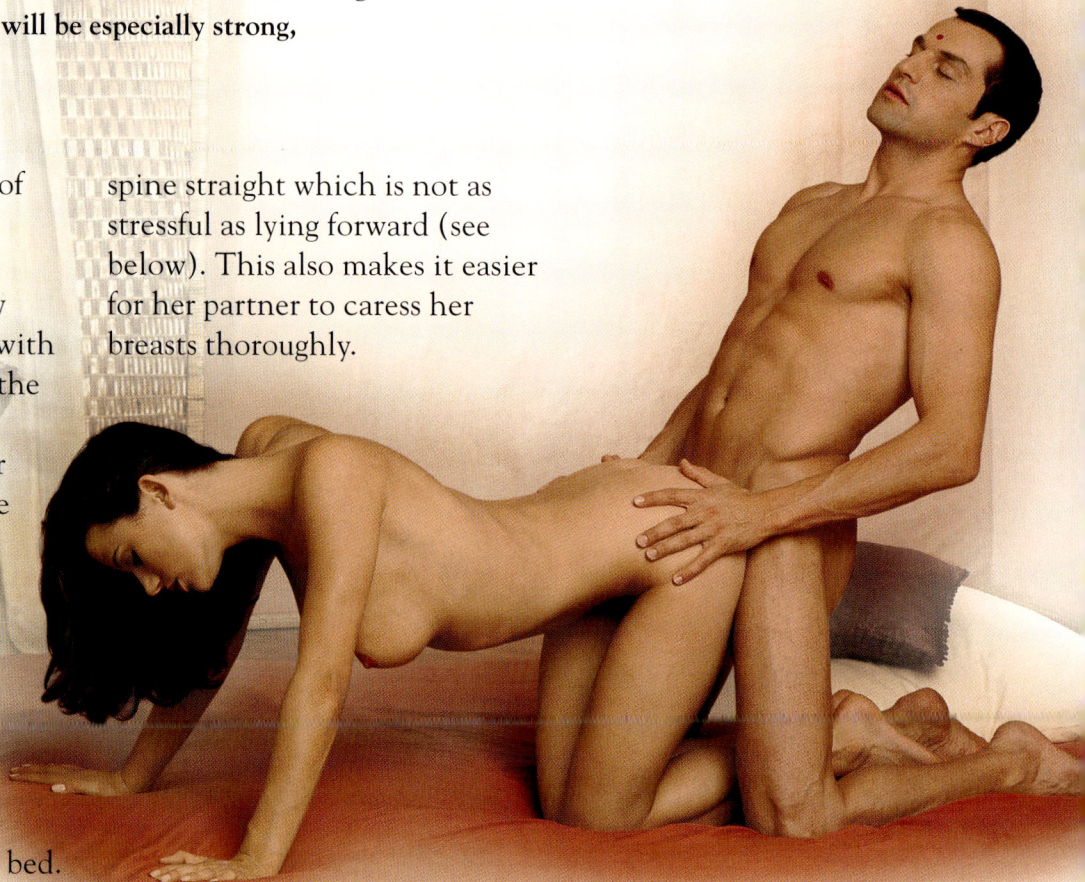

A variation of the Tiger position. Each partner feels the other intensely.

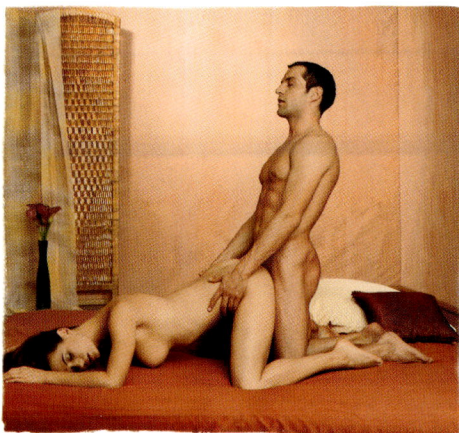

Open Tiger Position

This posture is similar to the Closed Tiger in that the woman kneels in front of her partner, but this time the woman has her legs spread apart. While her head and upper body lean for-

Deep penetration is possible with the Open Tiger position.

ward, the woman raises her pelvis and backside as high as possible to signal her desire as well as absolute devotion. The man kneels behind her with his legs nearly closed. In this position Shiva is able to gently caress the back and buttocks of his lover.

Open Elephant Position

This position, called *gajasava* in Sanskrit, shows the woman lying on her abdomen with her legs parted and her head turned to the side. This may be made more comfortable if a pillow is placed beneath her pelvis so that her

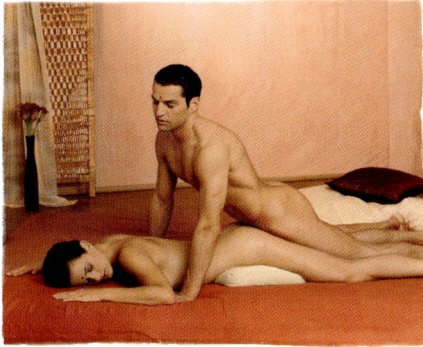

This position allows the woman to abandon herself to pleasure.

hips are a bit raised. The man can lie either in between her legs, supporting the weight of his body with his hands or elbows, or directly on her back, entering her from behind.

Love Swallow

The man sits on his heels while his partner lies with her pelvis in his lap, her legs around his hips, and her backside touching his abdomen. She should support her upper body with her hands, pushing her pelvis as far back as possible to enable penetration by her partner. The Love Swallow is only for men who have large penises and strong erections.

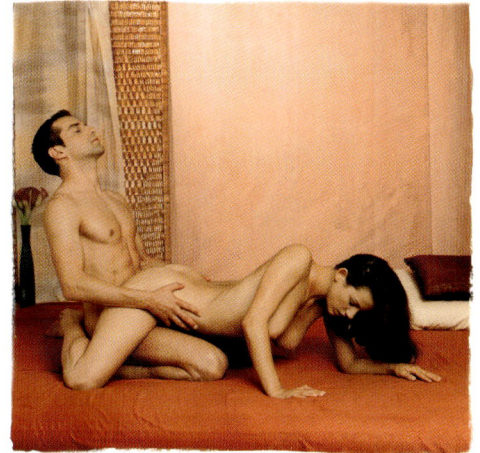

There are many variations of this position, which allow the male to caress and stroke his partner.

Closed Elephant Position

The beginning posture is the same as in the Open Elephant. After the lingam has penetrated the yoni of his Shakti, she brings her legs together while her partner spreads his; then both partners can extend their legs if they choose. In the Closed Elephant, genital stimulation is strongly felt by both the man and woman and the Shiva's erection can be maintained for a longer time.

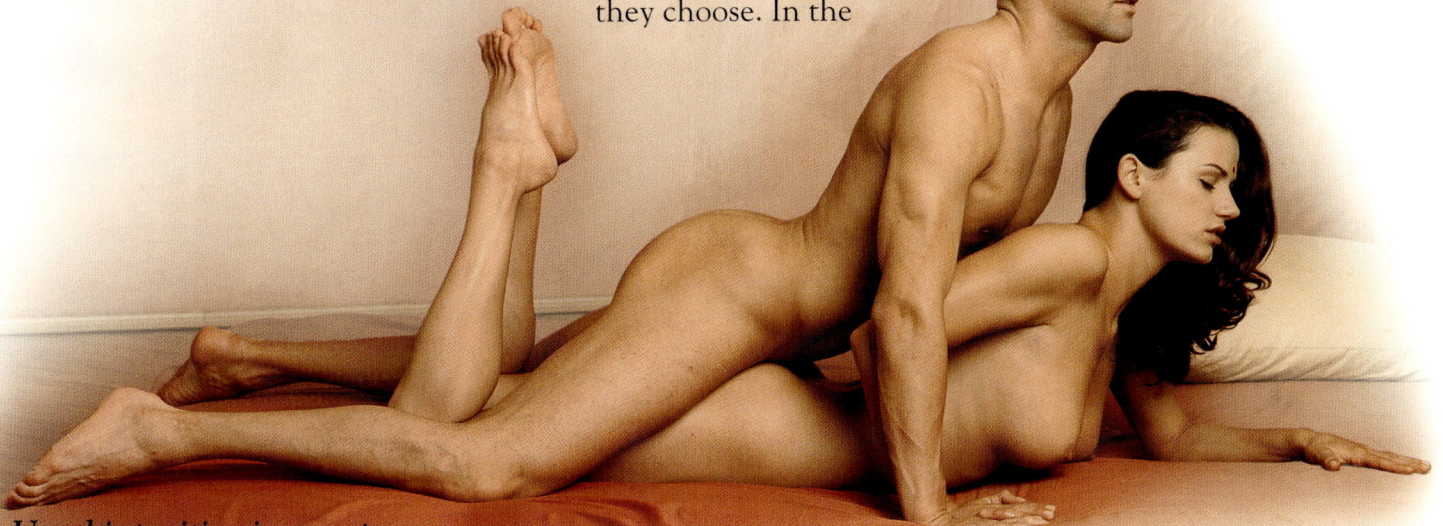

Use this position in an especially long game of love.

Sawana

In *sawana* positions, the man lies on his back and enjoys the passionate attention of his partner. The woman lies or sits astride him and controls the speed, intensity, and rhythm of intercourse.

The Forward Rider

In the *bhamra asana* position, the man reclines on his back with his legs together. His partner sits astride him with a knee on either side of his hips, then she directs his lingam into her yoni. She leans all the way forward so that her breasts touch his chest. In this as well as the following postures, the woman takes the initiative and controls the rhythm and depth of the thrusts.

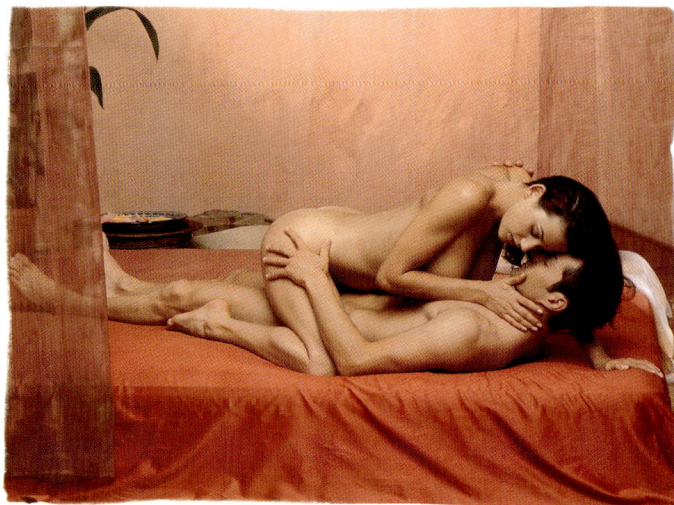

During love play in this position, enjoy the close contact between skin, and the eye contact.

Many men enjoy experiencing their partner's desire in this way.

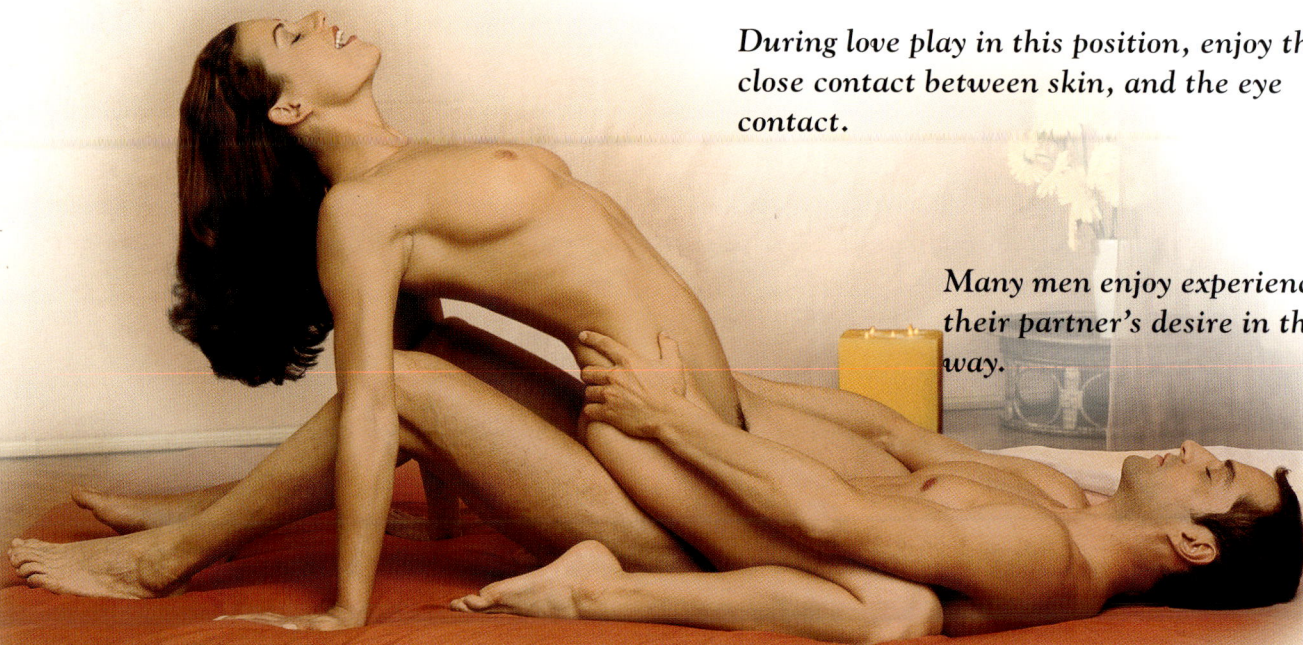

The Upright Rider

The position is the same as the Forward Rider (see above), but here the woman's upper body is erect or even leaning slightly backward, supported by her hands. Different variations have Shakti either kneeling over or sitting on her partner, with legs pressed together or crossed. Whichever she chooses, she should take the active role in making her partner feel aroused.

Crab Position

In this position, the woman sits or kneels turned around on her partner so her back is to him and she is facing his feet. Depending on how deeply and at what angle the lingam is able to enter the yoni, Shakti can either sit erect or lean backward to facilitate penetration.

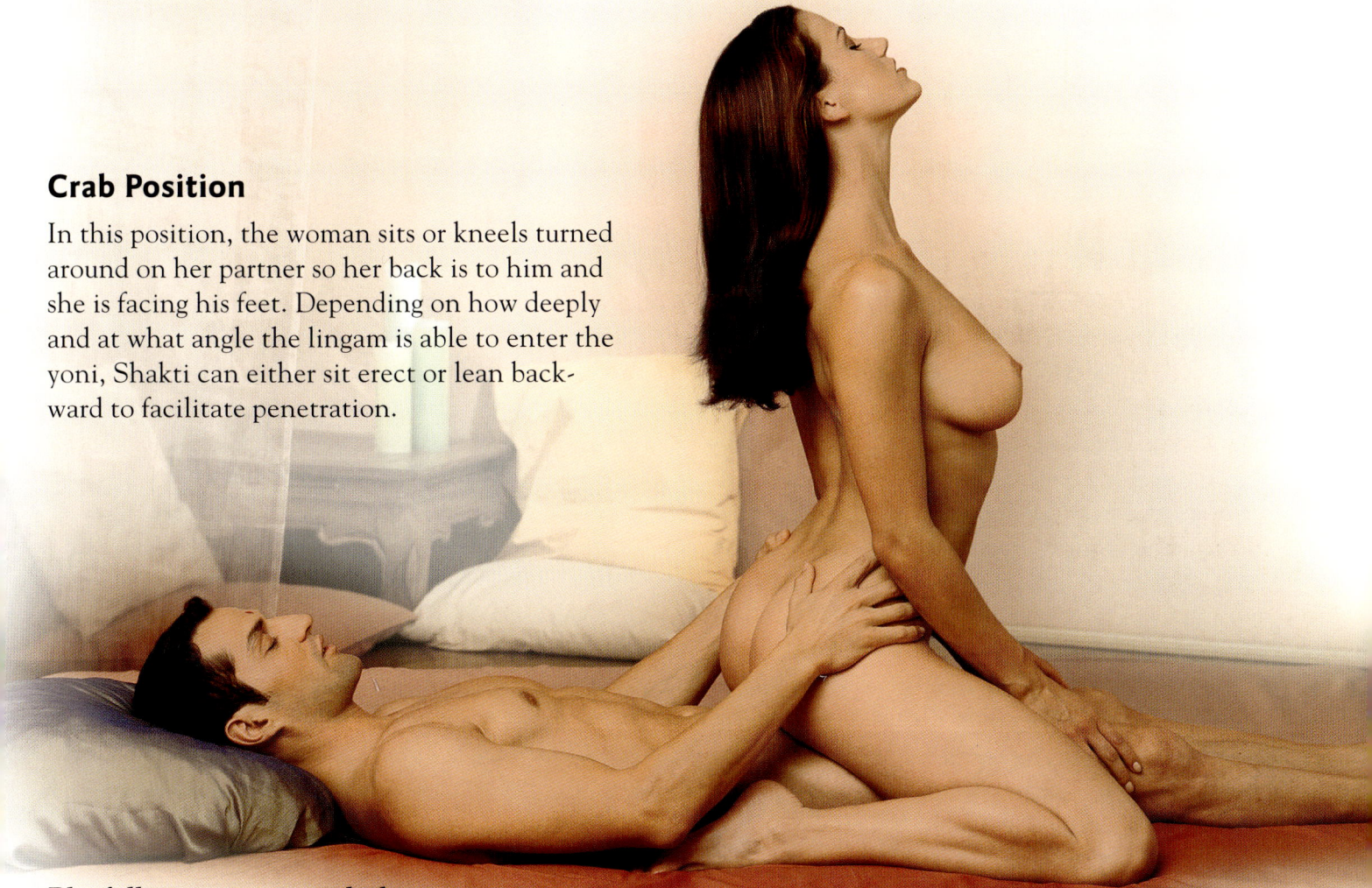

Playfully experiment with this position and see how arousing it is for both partners.

The Shakti Crouch

The man lies passively on his back with his legs together. His partner stands over him with legs placed on either side of his waist. She then crouches down over him deep enough so that she can insert his erect penis into her vagina. From this position, she is able to easily move up and down on top of him. She should balance herself by placing her hands on his shoulders while her partner holds her thighs.

The woman controls movement while her partner lies back and enjoys.

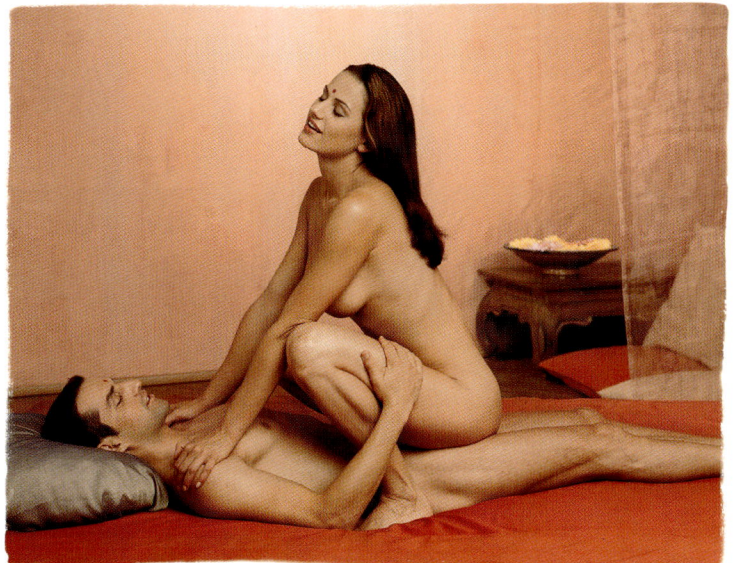

Conscious Control of Orgasm

Tantra is not about the quick satisfaction of lust. Couples who practice Tantra generally take the entire night for their lovemaking because they understand that it is only possible to reach the highest peak of sexual intensity through a gradual heightening of desire. Women especially enjoy this approach because it corresponds very closely to female sexuality.

Most women respond only gradually to touch. When the first level of desire is reached, arousal then increases in a wave-like momentum that accentuates the sensitivity and reaction of the body. Sexual excitement may be slower to develop, but it remains for longer and can be returned to again and again. This explains why many women are able to experience multiple orgasms in the space of one evening. The sexual landscape of Shakti resembles a smooth chain of hills, which transform into high, mountainous peaks.

In contrast to this, the male orgasm looks like a rapid development of a large mountain. Upon reaching the peak, a man soon loses energy, becomes tired, and may even sleep soon afterward. This illustrates a man's quick reaction to sexual stimulus which results in quick orgasm, and the ebbing of desire immediately afterward. As can be seen, in regard to sex, men and women are not at all well synchronized. But Tantra has a solution—the control of male orgasm!

According to tantric theory, the source of female sexual energy is almost inexhaustible and requires no conservation while males should preserve their energy or, more specifically, ejaculation. Taoist Tantra suggests that men above the age of 35 should ejaculate once a month at most because storing the "elixir of life" leads to rejuvenation and surprising vitality. In the Tantra practiced in India, ejaculation during intercourse was allowed as long as it happened sparingly and not too quickly. The intent of these rules is not to torture men—quite the opposite. If a man is able to adjust his level of arousal to that of his partner, the culmination of the sexual act will be more pleasurable for both.

Masters of Tantra have the ability to engage in sexual intercourse for hours, to revive desire over and over again and, most importantly, to experience an orgasm that lasts several minutes. The secret lies in increasing sexual arousal until shortly before reaching the peak. As soon as a man recognizes that he is close to orgasm, he should ask his partner to remain motionless while he completely relaxes his thighs, backside, stomach, and pelvic floor muscles while performing the yoga complete breathing technique three times (see page 32). Alternately, he should chant the mantra *pa da omam* (inhale on the *pa da*, exhale on the *omam*) to himself several times and imagine a red beam of light rising from his pelvic floor toward his heart chakra.

The more a man practices this exercise—approaching the limits of orgasm, consciously relaxing, and then approaching the limits again—the easier it will be to prolong the sexual act and ultimately to experience very powerful orgasms.

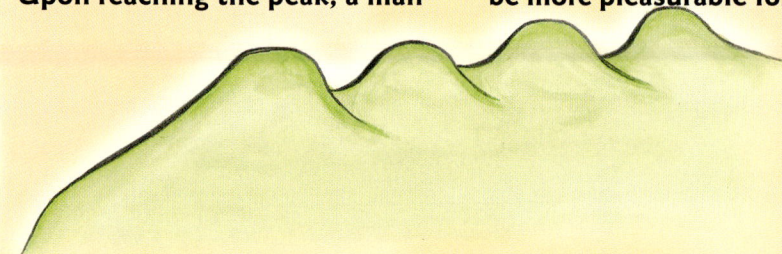

The female orgasm is composed of several smaller and larger waves of desire.

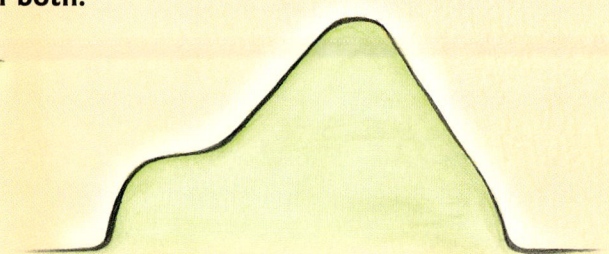

The level of excitement in a male rises quickly and results in only one orgasm.

Triyak

Positions in which both partners lie on their side facing each other are called *triyak* in Tantra. It is difficult to perform vigorous pelvic movements in such positions, but the couple can experience long and intimate intercourse instead.

Open Pearl Oyster

Both partners lie on their side facing each other. The man brings his legs together and puts them in between the open thighs of his lover, who then wraps her legs around his hips; one leg below and one over his body. (The Open Pearl Oyster should only be performed on a soft mattress, or Shakti's lower leg could become numb).

Variations

In this lateral position the leg positions may be exchanged. When her partner has entered her, the woman can then close her legs while the man opens his, laying one over her hips.

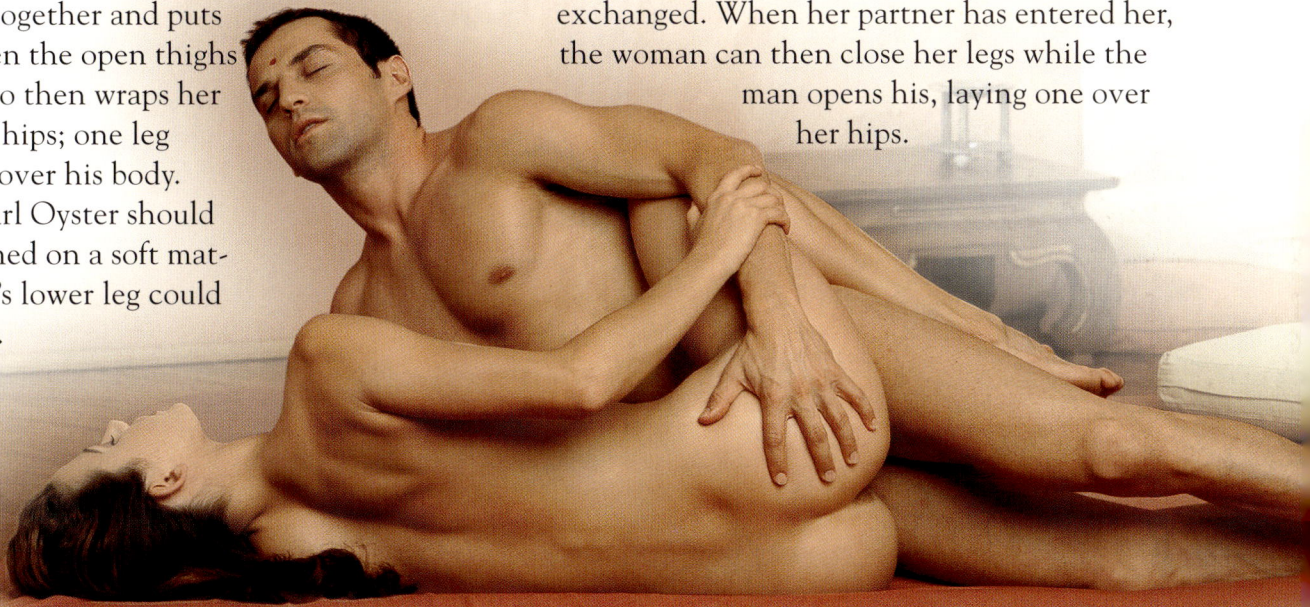

This position allows both partners to keep freedom of movement.

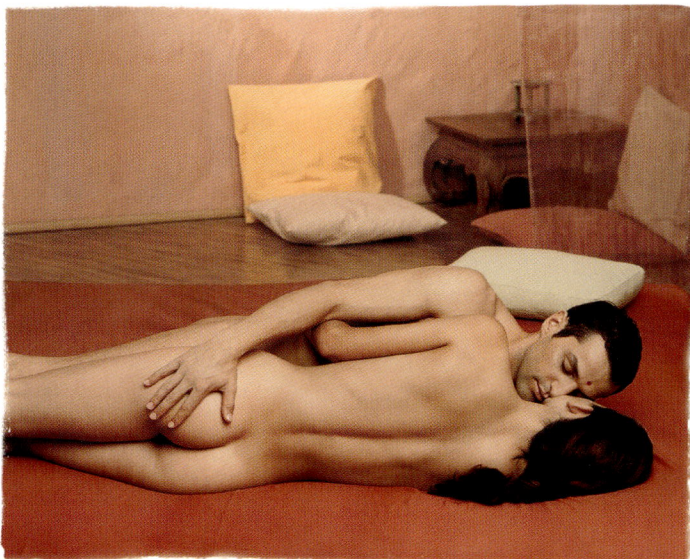

Closed Pearl Oyster

As before, both partners lie on their side and face each other, but now both close their legs after the man has penetrated the woman. This position creates a tight merging of the sexual organs and a strong transfer of chakra energy.

In a lateral position, both partners feel the intimacy of intercourse.

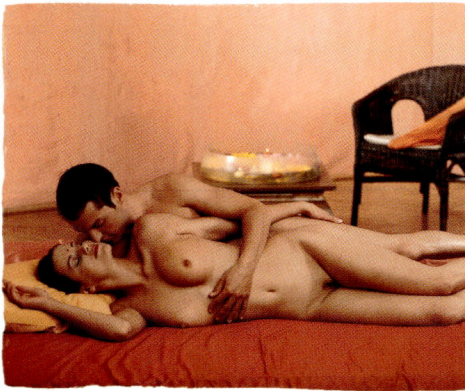

A sexual position that is comfortable for both partners.

Grotto Position

This position, also known as "spooning," also has both partners lying on their side, but now the man lies behind his Shakti with his chest and stomach pressed against her back. The woman should first open her legs to make penetration easier, then either let them remain open or close them again. The Grotto position allows Shiva to stroke the breasts of his partner or stimulate her labia and clitoris.

The Scissors

To get into position so that the man ends up lying on his side, the woman must first lie on her back with her legs drawn up. Her partner lies horizontally so that

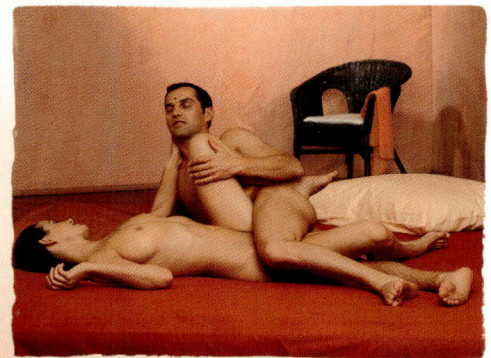

You can enjoy long acts of love in this position.

their torsos create a 90-degree angle. After her partner penetrates her, she extends her right leg, which the man covers with his left thigh. Then he moves his upper body next to his partner's so that she is able to place her left leg over his waist. The entwined legs are now scissored together.

The Dragonfly

In the Dragonfly only the woman lies on her side. The man must kneel behind her and penetrate her from behind. Shakti then extends her right leg and turns her upper body to the right so that her back touches the floor or bed, then bends her left leg. At the same time, her partner balances himself by raising his right leg and supports the extended leg of the woman with his left arm.

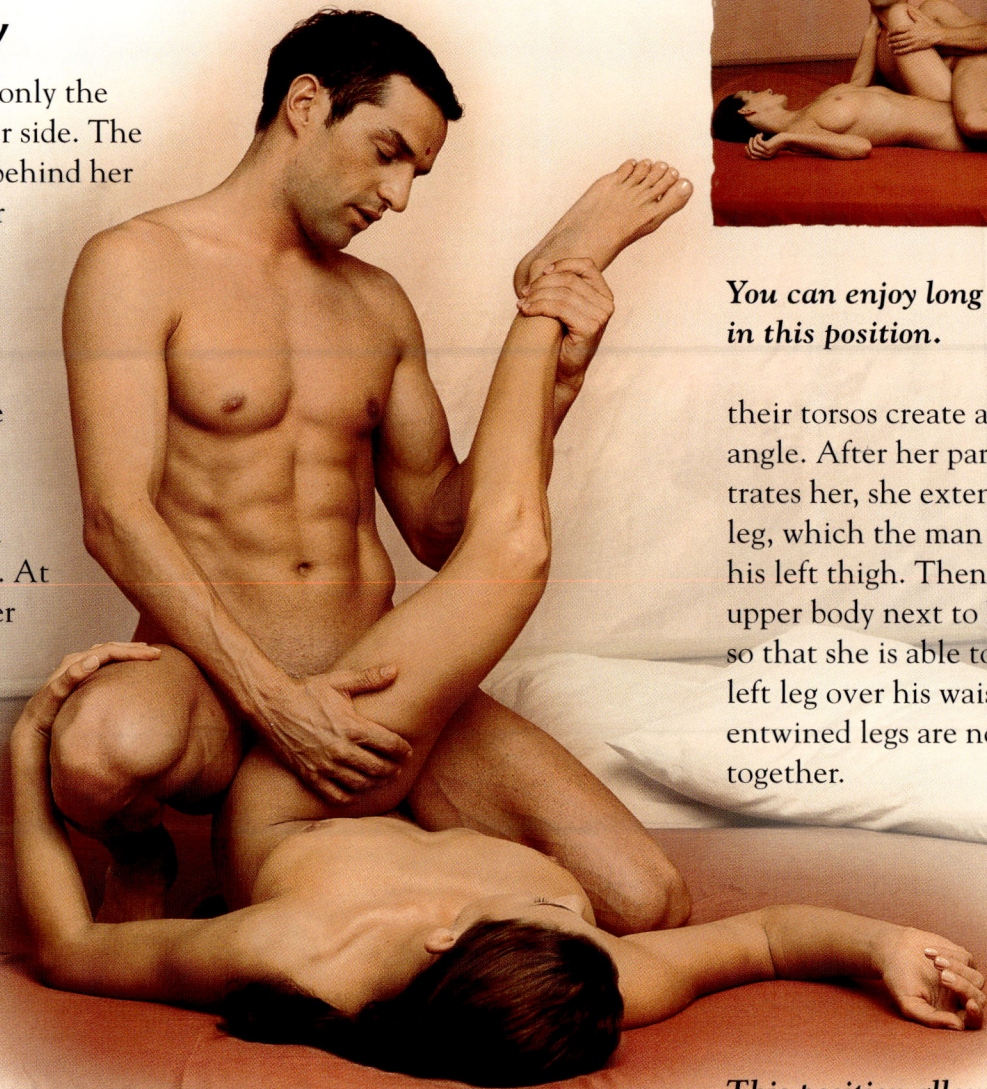

This position allows you to vary your love games.

Upavishta

Sitting positions, called *upavishta,* are very popular in Tantra because both partners experience the sexual act very consciously. Strong movements of the pelvis are not always possible, but these postures are very good for delaying orgasm, thereby prolonging intercourse.

Merging Lotus

All sitting positions are essentially variations of the Lotus position combining two people. These positions are very popular in Tantra, because the upright position of the spine promotes active engagement and awareness, and therefore enhances meditative merging.

For the traditional position *padma asana,* the knees and hip joints of the man need to be very flexible since he is seated in a modified Lotus position (half-lotus position, see page 30). He crosses his legs with the feet pulled into his body as close as possible. Because the posture is easier to perform if the pelvis is in a higher position, he should sit on a large pillow. Shakti sits on his lap with her legs around his waist and ankles crossed behind his back.

In this position, both partners experience active engagement in intercourse.

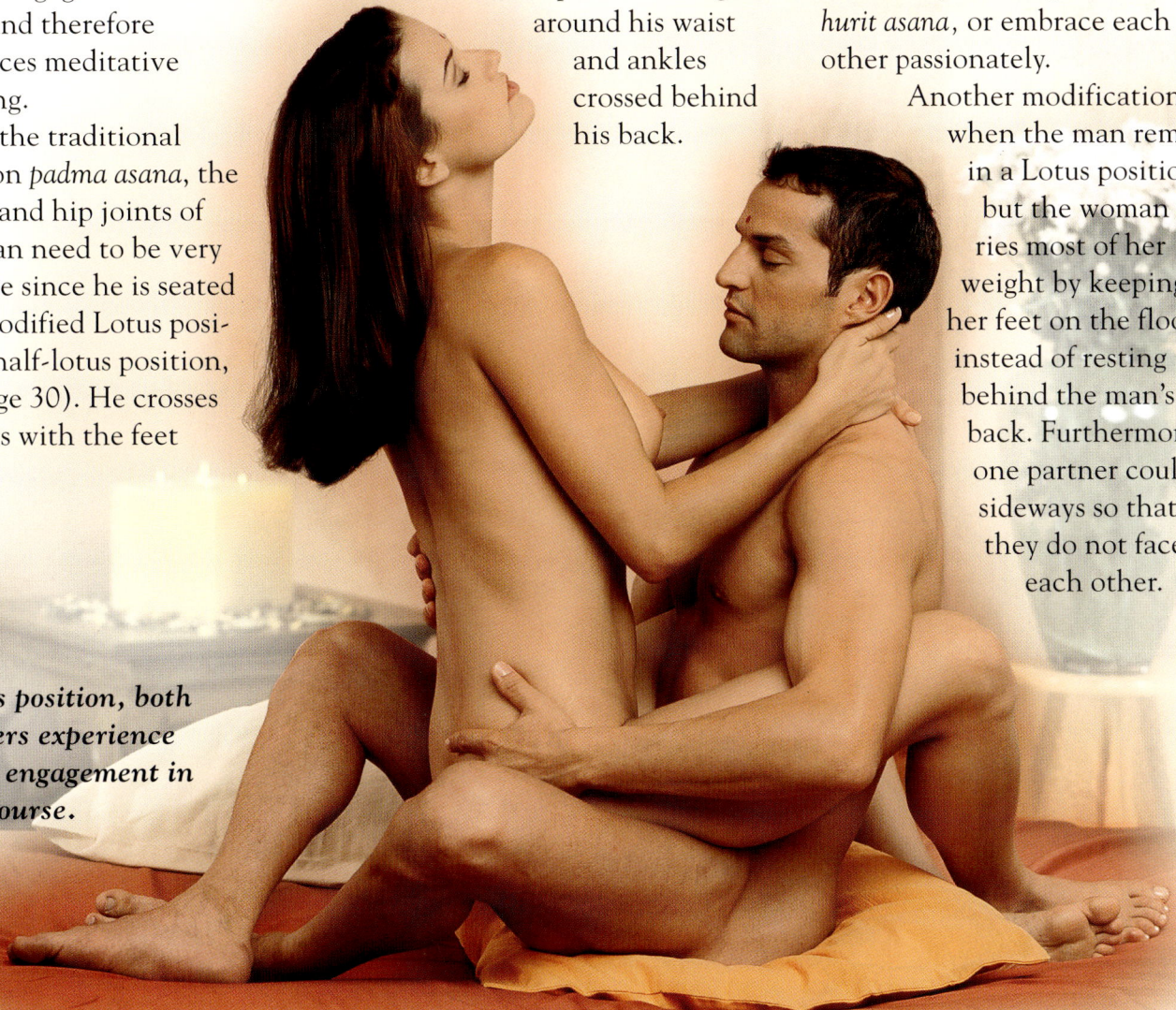

Variations

Sitting positions are much easier to maintain if the man sits cross-legged instead of in a Lotus position. The woman remains in the same posture as described above, and both partners perform *vaidhurit asana,* or embrace each other passionately.

Another modification is when the man remains in a Lotus position but the woman carries most of her weight by keeping her feet on the floor instead of resting behind the man's back. Furthermore, one partner could sit sideways so that they do not face each other.

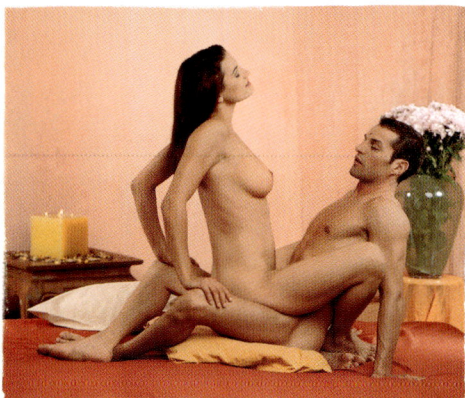

Both partners have the ability to move their pelvises in ways that give the other the most pleasure.

Supported Lotus

The man sits in a cross-legged position with his upper body leaning slightly backward. He supports himself by leaning on his arms, which are behind him. Shakti sits down on his erect penis, crosses her ankles behind his back, and supports her movements by pressing onto his thighs. In this manner, both partners have better agility in moving or rotating their pelvises.

The Lotus Swing

In the Lotus Swing, the man draws in his legs so he is able to place the soles of his feet together. His partner places her legs around his waist and crosses her ankles behind his back. This position, also called *sanyaman*, incorporates a swinging motion, which is possible when both partners have clasped their hands behind the other's neck. Leaning slightly backward, they then swing gently back and forth.

The Narrow Oyster

This sexual position is similar to the Wide Oyster (see next page), but the man should sit on his heels with his legs together. As the woman sits down on her partner's lap, she places her calves over the shoulders of Shiva, locks her ankles behind his neck, and supports her body by resting backward on her arms. The Narrow Oyster intensifies the contact between the penis and vagina.

Variation

If it is difficult for the man to remain sitting on his heels, he can either extend his legs outward or sit on the edge of the bed. The position of the woman does not change.

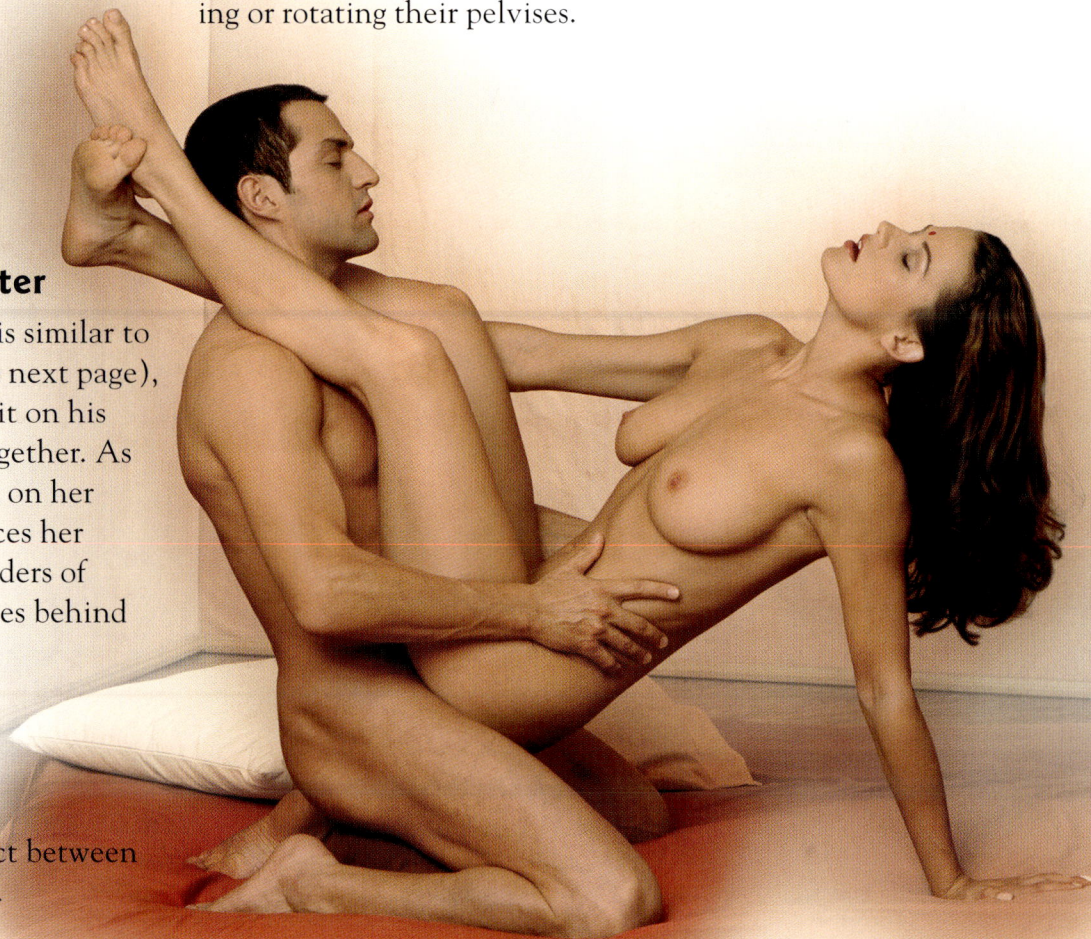

In the Narrow Oyster both partners feel the intense contact between lingam and yoni.

The V Position

In this position, Shiva sits on his heels with his legs open, and leans backward. His lover sits on his lap so that his lingam penetrates her. She then leans backward, supporting her weight with her arms, and extends her legs so that she can rest them on her partner's shoulders. Her posture should form the shape of a V. The angle in which the lingam rests in the yoni is pleasurable to both partners even though only minimal pelvic movements are possible.

If Shakti's stomach muscles are well trained, the couple can modify the position. The man can extend his legs so the woman sits between his thighs while she brings her legs close enough to her body that her thighs touch her breasts. This can be a very difficult position for the woman; therefore the

In this position, the slightest movement is felt.

man should hold her legs in order to stabilize them.

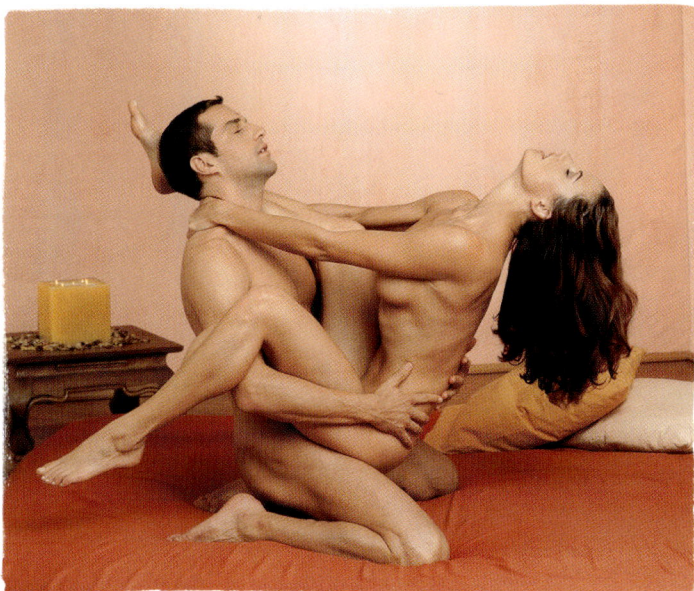

The Wide Oyster

The man sits on his heels with his legs slightly apart. His partner stands above him, then crouches so his lingam can enter her yoni. She clasps his neck and puts her legs around his waist while he holds her at the back or waist. Shakti then lifts her legs, keeping them wide open. The woman can also lean backward and support her weight with her hands.

The woman can either abandon herself to her partner or, supporting her own weight, share the active role.

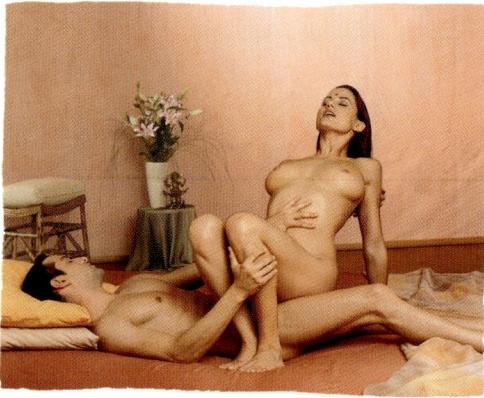

Shakti can direct the movements while Shiva spoils her with tender caresses.

Seat of Desire

In this position, the man lies on his back with legs extended. It is suggested that a large pillow be placed under his back so that his upper body is slightly raised. His partner sits sideways on his lap, and allows his penis to enter her. Supporting her upper body with her hands, she sits as she would in a chair, and controls the movement of the act.

The posture may be performed on the edge of a bed whereby the woman continues to support herself, but places her feet on the floor.

Twins Position

In the Twins position, both partners face the same direction. The man lies against a pillow with his legs stretched forward. His partner crouches over him, sitting on his lingam in such a way that her back faces him. Knees together, she leans backward over his body, supporting her weight with her arms. This position allows the man to stroke the breasts of his partner or massage her clitoris. To modify the position, the man should cross his legs or the woman should widen hers.

Kneeling Twins

This variation of the Twins position can be especially pleasurable for the woman. Since her

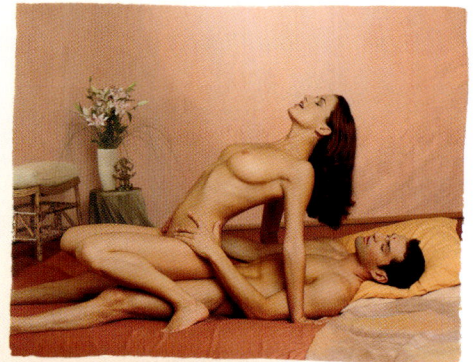

You can vary the Twins position according to your mood and desires.

partner has limited ability for movement, she directs the sexual act with rotations and pressure of her pelvis. The man sits on his heels while his partner sits on top of him with her back against his chest. By leaning forward or backward, Shakti can intensify her arousal.

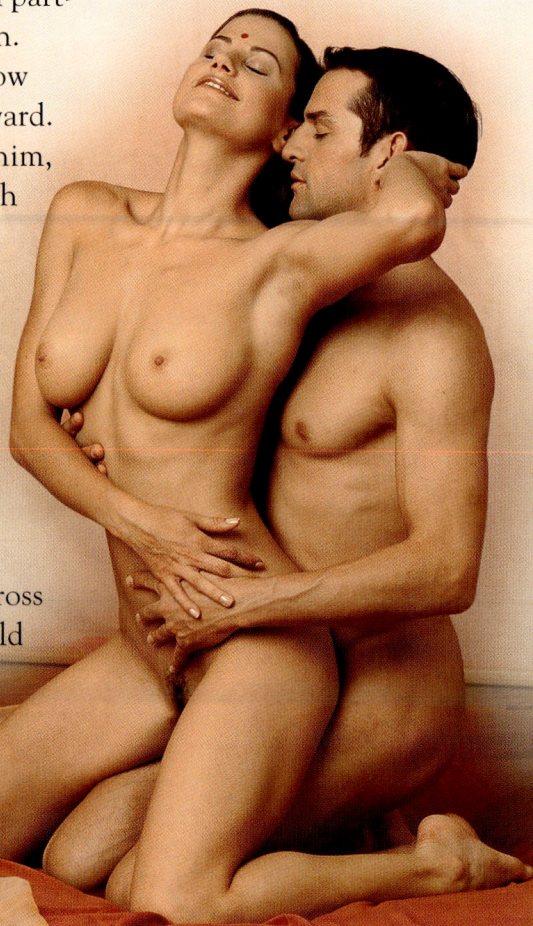

Shiva can further arouse his partner by gently stroking her body.

Uttita Bandha

Standing sexual positions can add a little variety to your love life. Some of them are fairly strenuous, but there are many other *uttita bandhas* that can be performed for a longer time.

Triangle Position

This sexual position, also known as the cow, finds the woman standing with her back facing her partner. Slightly parting her legs, she bends down far enough to grasp her shins or ankles. Her Shiva stands behind her and spreads his legs wide enough so that he can penetrate her grotto of desire comfortably.

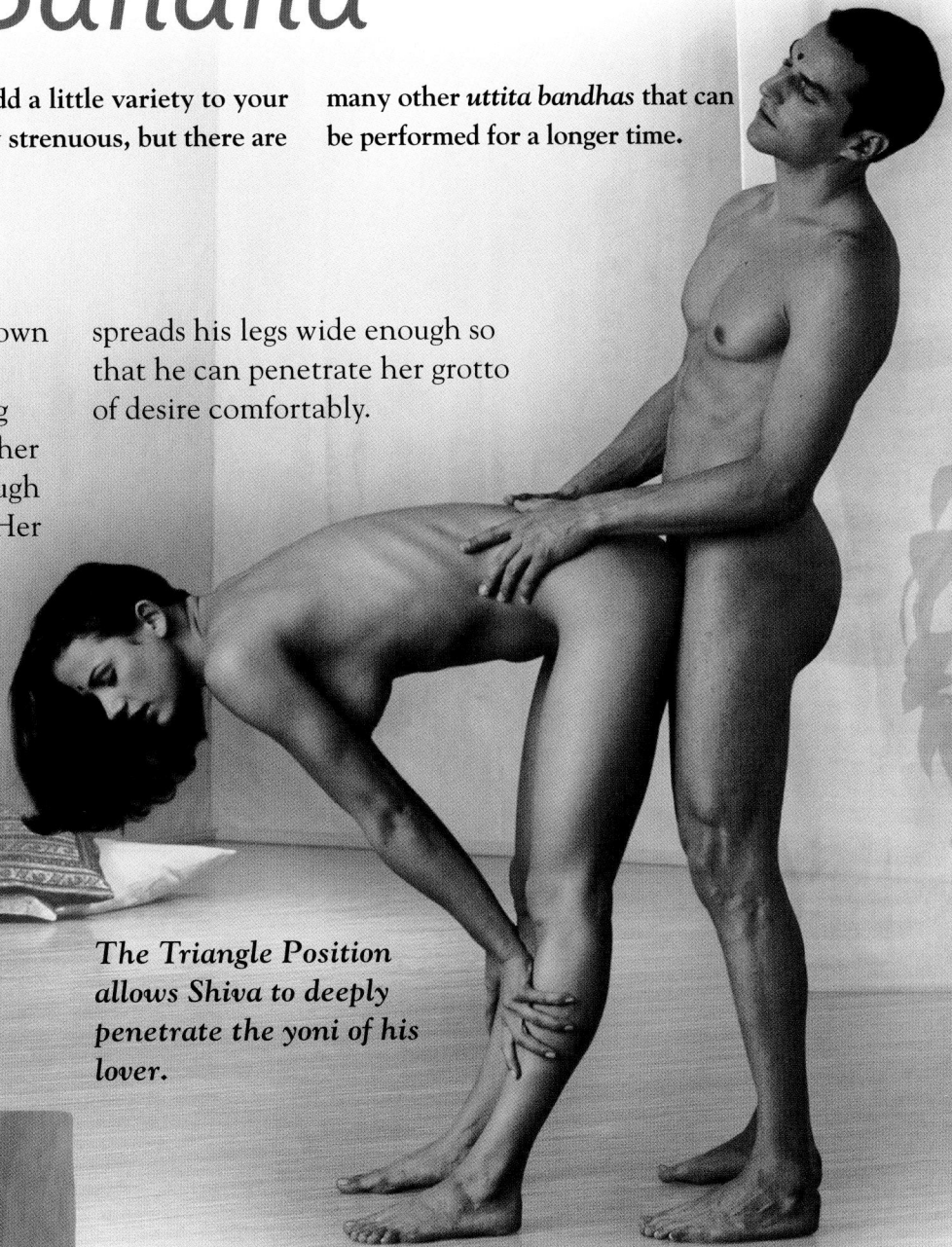

The Triangle Position allows Shiva to deeply penetrate the yoni of his lover.

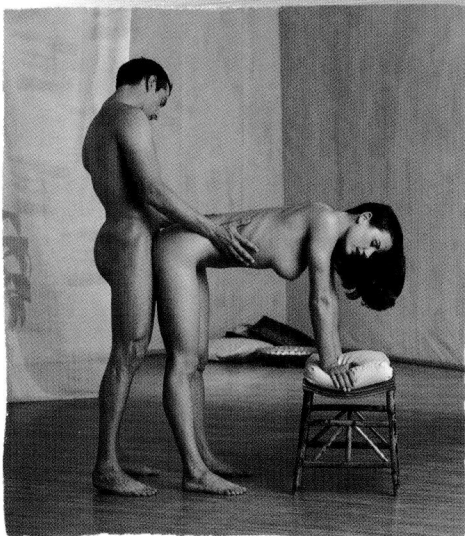

The Supported Triangle

This is a modification of the Triangle position that is easier to perform for the less agile Shakti who would not be able to bend so far forward. Again, the woman stands before her partner with her back facing him, but now she supports herself with the help of a stool, chair back, or edge of the bed when she bends over. Her legs are slightly parted and her back remains horizontal.

The man has the more active role in this position.

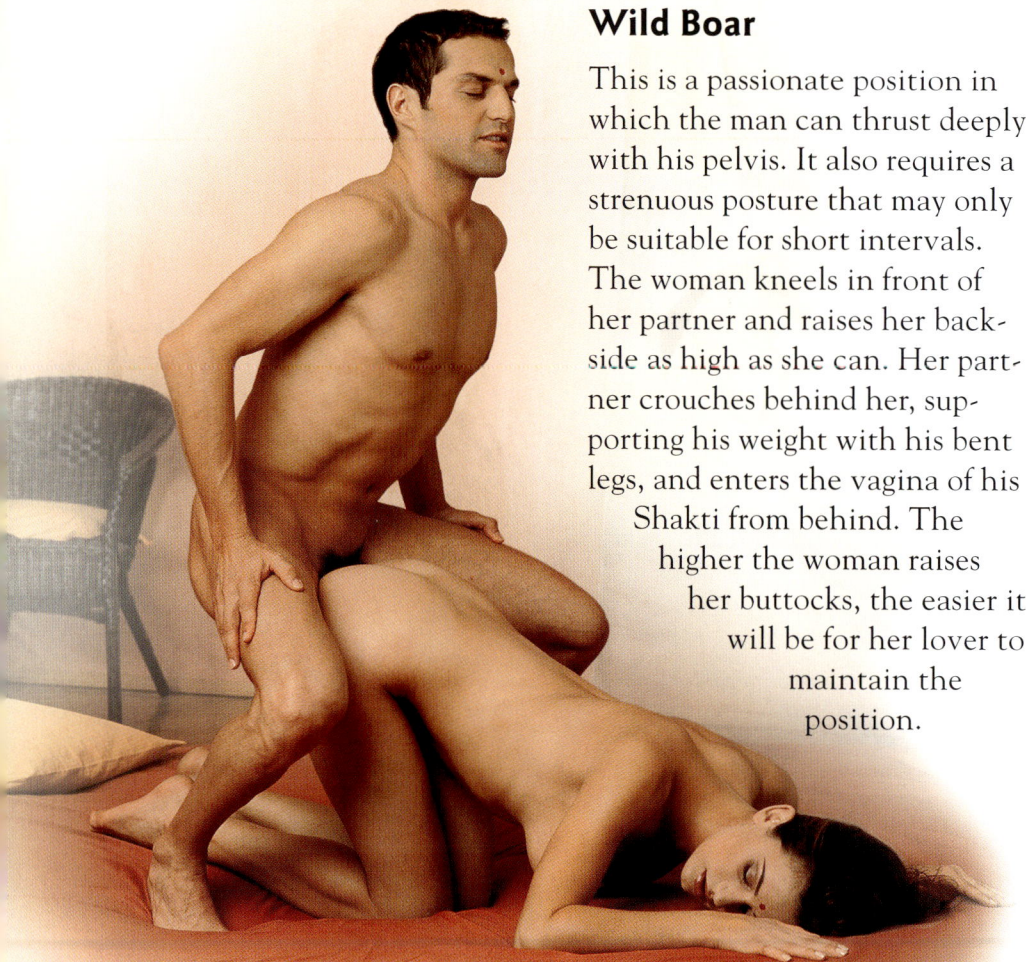

This position can be especially arousing for both partners.

Wild Boar

This is a passionate position in which the man can thrust deeply with his pelvis. It also requires a strenuous posture that may only be suitable for short intervals. The woman kneels in front of her partner and raises her backside as high as she can. Her partner crouches behind her, supporting his weight with his bent legs, and enters the vagina of his Shakti from behind. The higher the woman raises her buttocks, the easier it will be for her lover to maintain the position.

Wheelbarrow

The Wheelbarrow is for people who like to experiment. In India it was known as *manu ambhua* and used to show exceptional acrobatic ability in group rituals. To begin, the woman kneels in front of her partner with her hands placed firmly in front of her. Her partner stands behind her and, by grasping her ankles, lifts her pelvis high enough in order to penetrate her. Athletic couples usually find it easier to accomplish this posture since the woman must support most of her weight with her arms and also keep her thighs tense. The man must be able to hold her and also control movement.

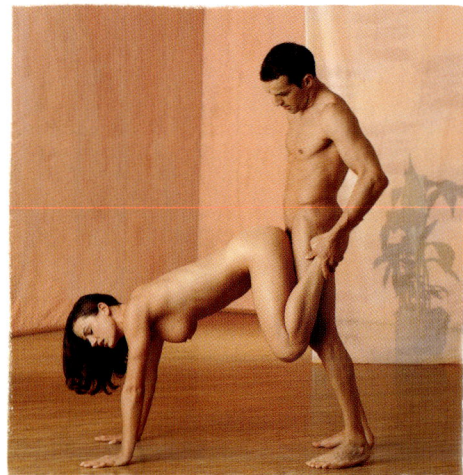

This position will certainly bring a change to your love life.

Love Hold

Because the man must carry the weight of his partner, the Love Hold is better suited to a stronger individual who has a light partner.

Shiva stands with his legs parted and knees slightly bent. His partner holds on to his neck with both hands, and then swings her legs around his waist. By crossing her calves over his backside, she can help to make this position easier for her lover. The man should grab the buttocks of his Shakti in order to both support her and to direct the movements of his pelvis. The Love Hold will be much easier if the man leans against a wall.

Variations

Variations of the position rely on the placement of the man's hands and arms. Instead of supporting his lover's backside, he may hold her ankles or place his lower arms below her knees and balance her against a wall.

Entwined Ivy

The man stands upright with his legs slightly parted. If the woman is much shorter, she may want to stand on a stool or chair. When she is nestled against him, her partner wraps one arm around her hips and loops one leg around his hip. In order to stabilize the position, the man should support the entwined leg against his hip with his free hand.

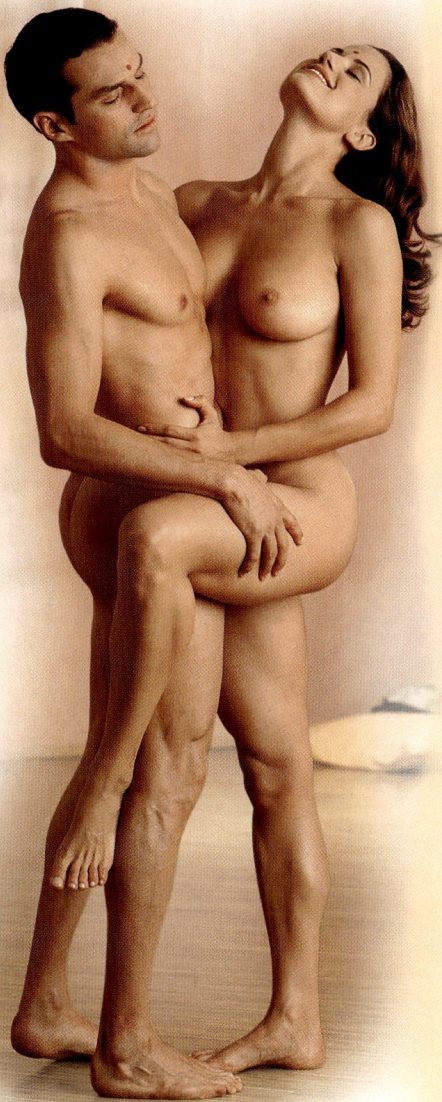

This position is suitable for couples who are nearly the same height.

The Art of Kissing

Tantra describes the many different techniques of kissing, including kisses on the lips, cheeks, neck, breasts, and the area in between the breasts. In India, it was believed that the souls were unified through a kiss and so the kiss plays an important role during, but especially prior to, sexual intercourse.

The most important kisses are considered to be:

🌀 The breathy kiss, in which the lips touch each other lightly

🌀 The pressure kiss, where the lips of the partner are moistened by the tip of the tongue

🌀 The sucking kiss, in which the upper or lower lip of the partner is sucked in and held

🌀 The exploring kiss, in which the tongue and mouth of the partner are explored with the kisser's tongue

🌀 The devouring kiss, in which both partners embrace passionately while kissing with their lips or tongues

Along with kissing techniques, Tantra considers the love bite as a means of arousal. Naturally, these are really gentle nibbles—although some Tantra couples do prefer painful biting in their games of arousal.

The following biting techniques are considered the most important:

🌀 The mosquito bite, in which the partner is gently nibbled with the incisors

🌀 The swelling bite, in which the lower lip of the partner is so strongly sucked that a blue swelling can appear

🌀 The half moon bite, through which a round imprint of the mouth is left on the partner's cheek

🌀 The pearl necklace bite, whereby little bites made with both the teeth and lips leave little marks that look like a necklace

🌀 The passionate storm kiss uses all the teeth and is used mostly in the breast area, but also on the backside and thighs

🌀 The bite of a boar uses the incisors and leaves little reddish marks on the shoulders, neck, and breasts

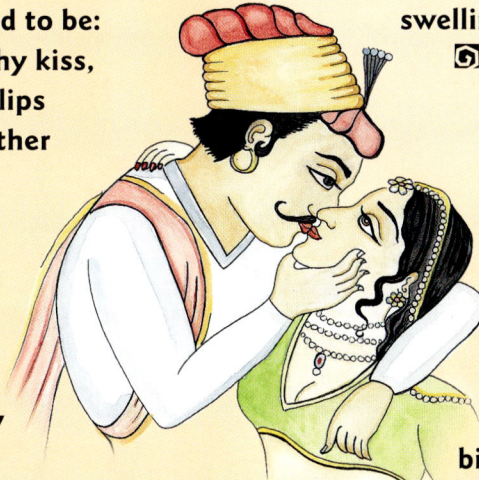

Aphrodisiacs

All agents that help increase sex drive are known as aphrodisiacs. The substances have been studied and used by all cultures throughout history and have also been utilized by followers of Tantra who were interested in stimulating arousal or prolonging erection. In contrast to earlier aphrodisiac recipes, which included animal parts such as pulverized rhinoceros horn, snake blood, monkey testicles, or even Spanish fly (a type of oil beetle), today's stimulants are made of plants containing substances that create an erotic tingling sensation. These are not only more aesthetic, they are also much more effective.

Viagra The pharmaceutical industry has developed its own aphrodisiac. The drug Viagra was originally developed to combat high blood pressure and angina, but was discovered to have much more success as a potency pill; it may be the best known chemically produced agent for sex. Although side effects are rare, some problems (and even deaths due to improper usage) have been reported. Therefore, all men should consult with their doctors and have a medical exam before taking this drug.

Those who study Tantra, however, have no need of chemical enhancers such as Viagra! Tantra-Yoga, breathing techniques, and sensual exercises, supplemented perhaps with natural plant extracts, will make it possible for men and women to enjoy all the pleasures of love until a very old age.

Expansion of Consciousness
Along with roots, herbs, and spices, mind-altering substances such as marijuana and alcohol have been used in Tantra with the specific purpose of expanding consciousness and intensifying intercourse between Shiva and Shakti. With that goal in mind, experimentation and careful observation of drug effects is a prerequisite to taking any.

The following pages will introduce you to the most important sexually stimulating substances. None of these are against the law and many are readily available.

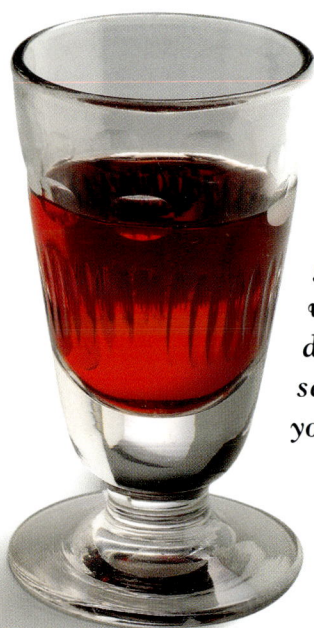

The first glass of red wine arouses desire; the second makes you sleepy.

The Best Ingredients from a Natural-Food Store

Many of these substances may seem boring. They do not contain exotic substances like animal testicles, blood, or crushed antler, but they are plants that contain very exciting medicinal properties.

There are very simple and obvious aphrodisiacs: we have seen that spices such as vanilla, chili, pepper, or celery seed can cause small miracles. Also, essential oils such as jasmine, rose, sandalwood, ylang-ylang, and patchouli stimulate sexual desire when used in a sensual manner; for example, in a sensual massage or vaporized in an aroma lamp (see page 60). Yet, a cup of coffee or a glass of red wine can also help awaken new life and desire.

Alcohol

Alcohol may be one of the oldest drugs known to mankind. The Sumerians, for example, were brewing beer 4,000 years ago, and the use of alcohol to stimulate libido has existed for centuries, if not thousands of years. Tantra has incorporated alcohol in the form of wine into its rituals.

For alcohol to be stimulating rather than soporific much depends on the quantity. In this case, less is more!

If you are drunk, you will not be able to practice Tantra! For men, 12 ounces of wine should be absolutely enough to produce a free and stimulating effect; women require even less! According to a 1994 study published in the science magazine *Nature*, testosterone production in women is increased through alcohol intake, leading to a significant increase in libido.

Alstonia (Alstonia scholaris)

Alstonia, also known as Australian fever bush, devil tree, fever bark, and Pali-mara, grows mainly in the tropical forests of East Asia and India. The seeds of the tree have been taken as a supplement to Tantra-Yoga techniques to strengthen the genital musculature. These seeds also contain alkaloid chlorogenin, which can cause mild irritation

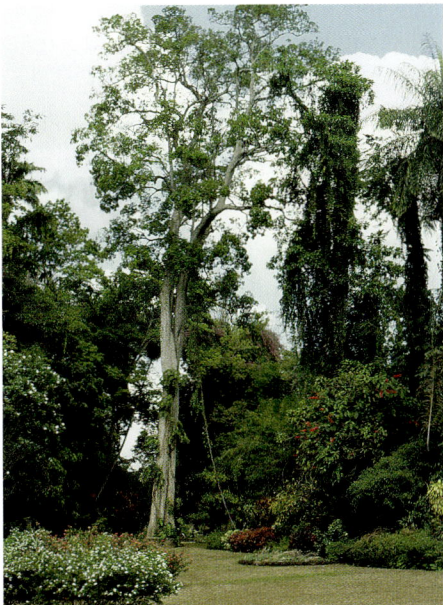

The devil tree, also known as fever bark, promises a long lasting erection.

of the urogenital tract, but the greatest effect is increased blood circulation and a tingling stimulation of the nerves, which causes a longer-lasting erection. This makes it possible to delay orgasm.

If you want to prepare the extract yourself, crush two grams of seeds in a mortar and then pour 16 ounces of water over it. Let this mixture sit for about twelve hours, then strain the water. Be sure to carefully experiment with the dosage; an overdose can cause irritation in the bladder and genitals.

Fo-Ti-Tieng (Hydrocotyle asiatica)

This plant, also known as gotu kola, originates in Asia. *fo-ti-tieng* is a Chinese name that means "elixir of long lasting life." In fact, scientists have discovered alkaloids in the plant which have been used for over a thousand years in China. These alkaloids have both detoxifying properties and also rejuvenating effects on the nerves, the brain, and glands of the endocrine system. Asians suggest drinking one cup daily to clean and revitalize the body.

For regular use, pour a cup of boiling water over half a teaspoon of ground leaves. Cover, and let brew for six minutes. The tea is used to strengthen nerves, the immune system, and digestion. To stimulate sexual energy, you

will require a higher dose—approximately two teaspoons of leaves for a large cup. Use this larger dosage for special occasions only.

Ginseng (Panax ginseng)

Ginseng grows in the deciduous forests of Korea and China, where the root has been regarded as a medicinal stimulant for over 5,000 years. Even today many Chinese doctors recommend daily usage of this magical root to improve health, life, and love. The healing effects of ginseng have been scientifically proven, and ginseng preparations are available almost everywhere.

Along with trace elements and vitamin B, ginseng contains saponine, a glucoside that stimulates the endocrine gland system, metabolism, blood circulation to the heart, and generally harmonizes the body. Ginseng tea and elixirs strengthen the production

Ginseng, with its forklike, spiky branches, is one of the most important medical herbs. It needs to grow at least ten years to develop its powerful effects.

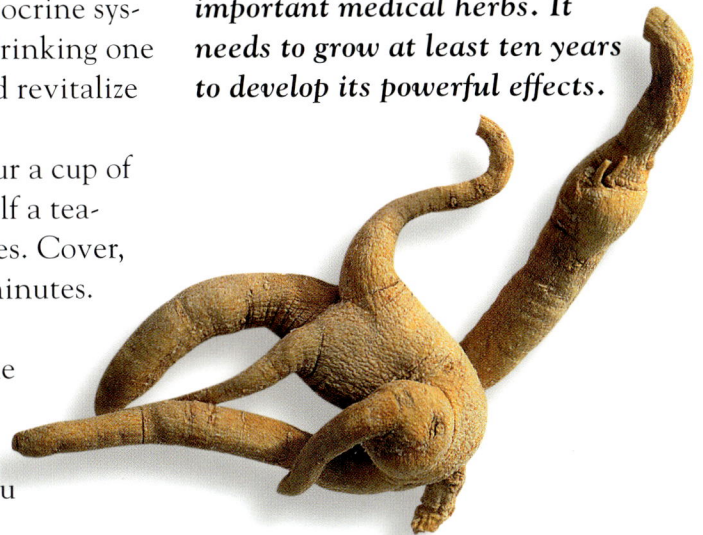

of sexual hormones and increase vitality, but only if used daily over a long period of time!

Guarana (Paullinia cupana)

Tribes indigenous to the rain forest have used Guarana for centuries. It has been used as a replacement for food in times of hunger, a treatment to combat poor digestion, and also an aphrodisiac. The rain forest vine, also known as the Brazilian cocoa tree, grows mainly in the rain forests of South America. Guarana itself is enclosed within a chestnutlike seed and must be dried before use. The substance contains approximately five times more caffeine than the coffee bean and is considered the

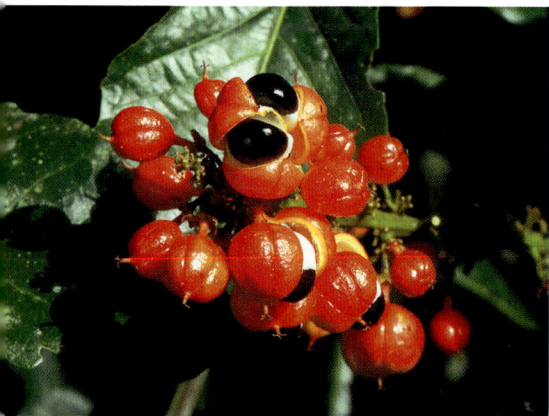

Guarana paste, a dark red-orange substance, is produced from seeds that have been dried and ground.

strongest of all the methylxanthines. Guarana stimulates the beating of the heart but at the same time has a relaxing effect on the vessels that assist in cre-

ating and maintaining an erection. Guarana powder is available in many health food and drug stores, but you can also crush the seeds yourself and prepare it as you would coffee. Use this sparingly—in excess it may cause insomnia and restlessness!

Ling Zhi-Pilz (Ganoderma lucidum)

Ling zhi-pilz is known in China as the godly fungus of the immortal. It is a rare fungus that is said to give eternal youth and lifelong joy in love. Today it is cultivated in large amounts in Japan and China, where it is then dried and shipped worldwide in the form of several compounds. Ling zhi-pilz is rich in polysaccharides, vitamins, triterpene, and amino acids. These compounds strengthen the immune system, aid in digestion, relax the nervous system, and stimulate genital organ functions. It also helps with potency and erectile problems, menstrual pain, and low sex drive. There are no known side effects.

Betel Nut (Areca catechu)

The betel nut is native to India and Southeast Asia, where the nuts ripen below the wide leaves of the Areca palm tree. In India, there is a very long tradition of chewing betel nuts. Frequent consumption causes the gums to turn a red color, which is much admired in Asia. The taste of the nut is improved when nutmeg,

cardamom, or paprika is added. It is often sold in combined form in markets.

The betel nut contains an alkaloid that has psychological effects, arecolin oil. This alkaloid stimulates the central nervous system: activates the salivary and sweat glands, decreases heart rate, and stimulates libido. If a pinch of burned lime is added to ground betel nut powder, arecolin oil can be absorbed through the mucous membrane of the mouth. This mixture should be kept in the mouth for at least a half hour before being spit out.

Caution Betel nut mixture should be taken only rarely, in small doses (1 gram), and should be chewed sparingly. Long-term use of this relatively aggressive mixture harms teeth and the mucous membrane of the mouth. Very strong overdoses (7–10 grams) can cause intoxication, diarrhea, and paralysis and even respiratory arrest, which may result in death! Consequently, the betel nut is rarely used in Tantra.

Glossary

Aphrodisiac (gr.-new lat.): Agent that stimulates sexual drive and increases desire (after the Greek goddess Aphrodite).

Asana (Sanskr.): Body position, posture, sexual position.

Bandha (Sanskr.): Clasp, knot, chain, or ribbon; further definition means Yoga techniques that store energy through the contraction of certain body parts.

Brahman (Sanskr.): Universal soul; Indian Vedic time, word spoken by high priests during sacrifices; later used as a religious-philosophical term describing the absolute principle.

Chakra (Sanskr.): Word for "wheel" or "vortex;" energy center of the astral bodies in the human body that absorb and store the energy of life (Prana).

Dakini (Sanskr.): Personification of the female energy principle; in Tantra, Dakini is venerated as both creator and destroyer; muse of eroticism and wisdom.

Ida (Sanskr.): One of the three most important energy paths in the astral body (see also Nadi); symbolizes female moon energy and runs from lower abdomen in a vertical line to the left side of the nose.

Kali (Sanskr.): From kala=time; wife of Shiva and mistress of time; she is omnipotent above all existence; she takes away fear and brings eternal freedom to her worshipers, who honor her with sexual rituals.

Kama Sutra (Sanskr.): Most famous of the main writings about the Indian art of love.

Krishna (Sanskr.): Worshiped in Hindu mythology as the eighth incarnation of the god Vishnu; shown as mostly blue; personifies male sexuality.

Kumbhaka (Sanskr.): Holding breath (from Sanskrit *kumbhak*, for container or pot); Yoga technique of holding the breath so that lower body transforms into shape of a pot.

Kundalini (Sanskr.): Snake power, power of the spiral (Sanskrit *kunda*, for pond or collecting basin); rests in the root chakra until awakened by special exercises, then rises through the central canal (*sushuma*) and connects with cosmic awareness.

Lingam (Sanskr.): Phallus; symbol of the god Shiva; cosmic principle of transcendence.

Mahakala (Sanskr.): One name of Shiva, meaning "great time;" Shiva as a tantric god who protects and guards the mysteries.

Maithuna (Sanskr.): Sexual intercourse in Tantra, either physical or symbolic.

Mantra (Sanskr.): Words or syllables with mystic power that concentrates the spirit through thought or spoken word; also used to control sexual energies.

Nadis (Sanskr.): Astral energy channels; Yoga writings describe 72,000 energy paths through the human body.

Parvati (Sanskr.): Companion of Shiva; symbol of the transcendental abundance and blissful happiness of tantric intercourse.

Prana (Sanskr.): Breath, life energy; astral energy that is absorbed primarily through breath; serves as a life energy for the cells and rests in the region of the heart.

Pranayama (Sanskr.): Literally "control of breath;" Yoga breathing exercises that lead to the conscious management of Prana.

Samadhi (Sanskr.): State of deep meditation where the duality between subject and object is abolished; dissolution of self in the cosmic order.

Shakti (Sanskr.): Godly wife of Shiva and sexual partner in ritual Tantra; generally known as the omnipotent female principle of creation.

Shiva (Sanskr.): Literally "the gracious"; one of the three main gods of Hinduism (along with Vishnu and Brahma); worshiped by some as the highest deity; personifies both creation and destruction.

Sushumna (Sanskr.): Central channel; main channel of astral love also called "path of Brahma" connecting the seven chakras with each other.

Tantra (Sanskr.): Thread, web; the Hindu Tantra is a group of religious texts describing the dialogue between Shiva and Parvati; discusses tantric rituals and principles and how sexual energy can be transformed into psychological energy, resulting in the awakening of kundalini; ritual of sexual intercourse that transforms into godlike merging.

Tantrica (Sanskr.): Followers of Tantra.

Upanishads (Sanskr.): To sit somewhere close (adore the master); mystical texts of Brahmanism; Vedic Upanishads written 200 to 400 years before the common era and including approximately 150 texts that deal with the personality of Brahma.

Veda (Sanskr.): Literally, knowledge; oldest religious literature of India; Veda consists of four collections of hymns that founded the Vedic religion and comprise part of the holy texts of Hinduism; four Vedas written in the earliest form of Sanskrit.

Yang (Chinese): The positive male principle containing qualities of light, strength, creation, heaven, movement, and rationality.

Yantra (Sanskr.): Mystical image in the form of a symbol or drawing; its purpose is to increase concentration and aid meditation.

Yin (Chinese): The negative female principle containing qualities of darkness, softness, tranquility, contemplation, comfort, earth, silence, and intuition.

Yoga (Sanskr.): Strain, harness, yoke (yoke from soul to God); exercises meant to transcend physical and mental limits in order to prepare for a state of contemplation; freedom from the deception of the senses and thoughts; conscious intercourse is the only true way to cosmic awareness.

Yoni (Sanskr.): Female genitalia; in India, the holy symbol of the female genitals.

INDEX

About the Author

Kalashatra Govinda was born in Bombay, India, in 1949, and has studied medicine and philosophy there. Beginning at age twelve, he studied the many schools of Yoga and was permitted to learn with some of the greatest yogis in India. After completing his studies, he became a professor and taught Kundalini-Yoga and Yoga philosophy at the University of Bangalore in South India.

All photography by Susanne Kracke, Munich (styling by Jacqueline Weber) with the exception of:
AKG Berlin: 10 (top), Jean-Louis Nou, 10 (bottom), 43, Werner Foreman;
A-Z Botanical Collection, London: 91 (left);
Ernst Beat, Basel (CH): 91 (right), 92;
Lance Dane, India: 14–15;
Photo Archive Steffens, Mainz: 16, 17 (top), Bridgman Art Library;
Südwest Verlag, Munich: 61 (bottom), Karl Newedel, 65 (background), Bernhardt Hecker, 90, Angela F. Endress

The material in this book was carefully researched and organized for the physical well-being and spiritual advancement of the reader. Readers with physical conditions of any kind should consult with a qualified health practitioner before ingesting any of the aphrodisiac preparations or attempting any of the exercises or positions suggested herein. Neither the author nor the publisher shall be held responsible for damage or discomfort that may result from the use of any information in this book.

Library of Congress Cataloging-in-Publication Data

Govinda, Kalashatra, 1949-
  Tantric ecstasy : the way of sacred sexuality / Kalashatra Govinda.
    p. cm.
Originally published in Germany under the title Tantra: Geheimnisse östlicher Liebeskunst.
  ISBN 1-4027-0057-1
  1. Sex—Religious aspects—Tantrism. 2. Sex instruction—Religious aspects—Tantrism. 3. Philosophy, Hindu. I. Title.
  HQ64 .G69 2003
  294.5'446—dc21

          2002155534

10 9 8 7 6 5 4 3 2 1

Published by Sterling Publishing Co., Inc.
387 Park Avenue South, New York, NY 10016
Originally published in Germany under the title *Tantra: Geheimnisse östlicher Liebeskunst* and © 2000 by W. Ludwig Buchverlag, Munich, Econ Ullstein List Verlag GmbH & Co KG, Munich 3. Edition 2001
English translation © 2003 by Sterling Publishing Co., Inc.
Distributed in Canada by Sterling Publishing
c/o Canadian Manda Group,
One Atlantic Avenue, Suite 105
Toronto, Ontario, Canada M6K 3E7
Distributed in Great Britain by Chrysalis Books
64 Brewery Road, London N7 9NT, England
Distributed in Australia by Capricorn Link (Australia) Pty. Ltd.
P.O. Box 704, Windsor, NSW 2756, Australia

Printed in China
All rights reserved

Sterling ISBN 1-4027-0057-1